THE GREAT BIRD FLU
HOAX

THE TRUTH THEY DON'T WANT YOU TO KNOW ABOUT THE "NEXT BIG PANDEMIC"

DR. JOSEPH MERCOLA
WITH PAM KILLEEN

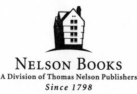

NELSON BOOKS
A Division of Thomas Nelson Publishers
Since 1798

www.thomasnelson.com

Published in Nashville, Tennessee, by Thomas Nelson, Inc.

Nelson Books titles may be purchased in bulk for educational, business, fundraising, or sales promotional use. For information, please e-mail SpecialMarkets@ThomasNelson.com.

ISBN 0-7852-2187-5

Printed in the United States of America

06 07 08 09 10 QW 5 4 3 2 1

CONTENTS

1. **The Plague That Never Was**   1
    What You Really Need to Know about the Bird Flu

2. **Sensation Sells**   29
    How and Why the Media Deceives You about
    the Bird Flu

3. **Bird Jails**   56
    Corporate Agribusiness and the Real Source of
    Bird-Borne Illness

4. **Shifting the Blame**   81
    How the Big Poultry Companies Make Money
    from the Bird Flu Scare

5. **Follow the Money**   99
    How the Drug Companies are Profiting from Fear

6. **Natural Cures**   124
    Improving Your Immune System to Protect
    Yourself from the Bird Flu

7. **A Silver Lining**   158
    Could the Bird Flu Be a Blessing in Disguise?

8. **Resources and Organizations to Help You**   195
    Stay Informed

Notes   215
Appendix   246
About the Author   250

1

THE PLAGUE THAT NEVER WAS

What You Really Need to Know about the Bird Flu

In 1918 children would skip rope to this rhyme:

> I had a little bird,
> Its name was Enza.
> I opened the window,
> And in-flu-enza.

Since 1997, when the first human contracted the highly pathogenic bird flu virus (H5N1) in Hong Kong, the disease has affected nearly fifty countries.[1] Bird flu has taken its toll in many areas of Asia, Africa, and Europe, killing 132 people as of the writing of this book. Millions of birds, both domestic and migratory, have also been killed as a result of the spread of this disease. To date, however, there hasn't even been one single reported case of the highly infectious bird flu in North America.

The title of this book, *The Great Bird Flu Hoax*, is not meant to suggest that the H5N1 virus does not exist, or that people have not died from this strain of the bird flu. The H5N1 virus is genuine, and the deaths it has caused are tragic and not to be disregarded or belittled in any way.

But after years of media-driven panic about the illness, only a relatively small number of people have been affected by it, compared to the millions of people who have died from many other acute and chronic diseases that genuinely threaten us today. The widely forecasted bird flu pandemic has not yet arrived, and as you will discover by reading this book, it is never going to arrive.

> **The widely forecasted bird flu pandemic has not yet arrived, and as you will discover by reading this book, it is never going to arrive.**

The bird flu "hoax" is the deliberately disproportionate attention the media and government are putting upon this specific infection in an attempt to frighten you about a nearly baseless threat. Once you understand the factors we review in the book, it will become quite clear that the motivation behind this media promotion is straightforward—there are a number of individuals and corporations that are profiting greatly from the frightened frenzy that is being created.

Before taking a closer look at those groups and their motives, first I'd like to tell you the information about the bird flu that you aren't being told—what it is, how far it has spread, and why, in all probability, you will never catch it.

What Is the Bird Flu?

The bird flu virus itself is nothing new; it's been around for ages. There are several strains of avian influenza, some of which have been shown to infect humans: these include viruses of the H5 subtype (H5N1), the H7 subtype (H7N2, H7N3, H7N7), the H9 subtype

(H9N2), and the H10 subtype (H10N7).[2] In total, there are 144 possible strains of the bird flu.

For many centuries, the bird flu has typically been a relatively minor illness even in birds. The recent appearance of the highly infectious bird flu strain H5N1 that has killed poultry and now people is a new phenomenon, and it is likely *not* due to some unfortunate and random genetic mutation. Rather, the occurrence of this more dangerous form of the virus coincides quite nicely with the increase of large poultry operations (factory farms) and transnational poultry production.[3] As I will explain in more detail later, the emergence of this highly infectious bird flu virus is closely related to the current practices of the poultry industry.

Many "experts" have blamed wild birds, rather than the primary culprit, factory farming practices, for the spread of the virus. Some have alleged that wild water fowl can act as hosts by carrying the virus in their intestines and shedding it in saliva, nasal secretions, and feces. But the viruses circulating in wild birds are generally not the highly pathogenic avian influenza strains (called HPAI viruses) that cause deadly bird flu; they are low pathogenic avian influenza (LPAI) viruses that often do not even cause symptoms in the birds themselves.

Highly infectious bird flu viruses can cause severe epidemics in domestic chickens. Infection can result in a wide spectrum of symptoms in birds, ranging from mild illness to a very contagious and rapidly fatal disease.[4, 5] Symptoms of the bird flu infection in humans can depend on the particular strain of virus.

Several outbreaks of different strains of avian flu have been identified in various countries around the world, almost always with no reported human deaths. While HPAI viruses such as H5N1 have not appeared in North America, one variant that is less infectious to humans, H7N2, has been found in poultry in eight states since 2001. In 2004, another similar strain (H7N3) was found in large poultry operations in British Columbia, Canada. As a result of these outbreaks, millions of poultry were killed in an attempt to stop the spread of the disease.[6]

Whenever a bird flu virus has been detected among poultry, millions of birds have typically been destroyed as a control measure intended to limit or halt the spread of the disease. As H5N1 has been found in Asia, Europe, the Middle East, and Africa, about 200 million birds have been sacrificed at the altar of disease prevention. One of the problems with this approach is that many, if not most, of the birds that are killed in this manner are not necessarily sick at all; they are simply considered to be "at risk." In addition to culling birds, in some cases vaccines have also been used as an extra measure to stop the reemergence of the virus.

If you're worried about "catching" the bird flu, it's important to note that most varieties are not fatal to humans; but more importantly, nearly all of those who have been infected with any strain, including the highly pathogenic H5N1 virus, have been in close contact with sick poultry. So if your circumstances don't bring you in close contact with sick birds, your risk for acquiring this infection is remote at best.

Generally, in cases of avian flu outbreaks that affect humans (H7N2, H7N3, or H7N7, for example), it is poultry workers who have become ill, and they usually only exhibit some flu-like symptoms or eye infections (conjunctivitis).[7] In 2002, during the H7N2 outbreak in Virginia, a government worker who was involved with destroying poultry suffered fever, a cough, a sore throat, and a headache.[8] In 2003, an H7N7 bird flu outbreak in the Netherlands mostly infected poultry workers, causing one death and some speculation that there may have been three possible instances of transmission from poultry workers to family members.[9]

MAJOR OUTBREAKS OF AVIAN INFLUENZA[10, 11,12]				
Year	Subtype	Location	Impact	Comments
1983	H5	Pennsylvania	Caused severe clinical disease and high mortality rates in chickens, turkeys, and guinea fowl. 17 million birds were culled.	A serologically identical but apparently mild virus had been circulating in poultry in the area for 6 months. No human cases were identified.
1994–2003	HRN2	Mexico	Nearly a billion birds have been affected.	An LPAI virus mutated to an HPAI virus and caused an outbreak in 1994–95. The HRN2 strain has continued to circulate in Mexico since that time. No human cases have been identified.
1995–2003	H7N3	Pakistan	About 3.2 million birds died from avian influenza during initial outbreak in 1995.	A vaccination campaign apparently ended the outbreak. No human cases were identified.
1997	H5N1	Hong Kong	Virus was isolated from chickens; avian mortality rates were high—1.5 million birds were culled in three days.	18 human cases with 6 deaths were recognized. Prior to this outbreak H5N1 was not known to infect humans.
2003	H7N7	The Netherlands	30 million birds out of 100 million birds in the country were killed; 255 flocks were infected. Disease spread to Belgium but was quite rapidly contained.	Over 80 human cases were reported and one veterinarian died. Most of the human cases involved conjunctivitis.

2003–2006 (ongoing)	H5N1	Asia, Europe, Africa	By far the most severe outbreak of avian influenza ever recognized. As of December 2005, over 140 million birds have died or been culled.	More than 200 human cases have been recognized, with more than half of them fatal, in Vietnam, Thailand, Cambodia, Indonesia, China, Turkey, Iraq, Egypt, Azerbaijan, Djibouti.
2004	H7N3	British Columbia	Over 19 million birds were culled.	Two human cases were recognized; both patients had conjunctivitis.
2005	H7	North Korea	About 200,000 birds culled as of April 2005.	No human cases have been identified.
*Additional outbreaks of HPAI have been identified in a variety of countries Adapted from Capua (2004)				

Reproduced with permission from Avian Influenza (BirdFlu): Agricultural and Wildlife considerations. Center for Infectious Disease Research & Policy, University of Minnesota. Last updated July 19, 2006, at http://www.cidrap.umn.edu/cidrap/content/influenza/biofacts/avflu.htm.

- Australia had outbreaks of HPAI in 1976 (H7N7), 1985 (H7N7), 1992 (H7N3), 1994 (H7N3), and 1997 (H7N4).

- Italy had outbreaks in 1997 (H5N2), 1998 (H5N9), 1999–2001 (H7N1), and 2002–2003 (H7N3).

- The Republic of Ireland had an outbreak in 1998 (H7N7) that spread into Northern Ireland as well.[13]

H5N1

The highly infectious H5N1 virus has been found in several countries, moving from the East (China), to the West (France), and into Africa. The World Health Organization (WHO) explains that humans who have been infected by the H5N1 virus demonstrate a variety of symptoms:

- High fever and influenza-like symptoms

- Diarrhea

- Vomiting

- Abdominal pain

- Chest pain

- Bleeding from the nose and gums

- Difficulty breathing

- Pneumonia[14]

As with all strains of bird flu, the majority of humans who have been infected with this form of the virus have been in close contact with sick poultry.[15] In a few cases, officials determined that the virus could have spread through human-to-human contact. In the majority of such cases, the people who were infected were in close proximity to each other.

Officials claim that they are concerned about this particular strain of the bird flu because it has killed over half of the infected victims. While this fatality rate would certainly be alarming if true, it is far from accurate. There is an important distinction to make. In *The New York Times* article "Bird Flu: A Less Deadly Disaster?" (March 16 2005), Lawrence K. Altman, M.D., mentions that for every person sick enough to seek treatment there are likely many others with a milder form who forego examination or testing, which skews the fatality statistics.

Why Did President Bush Cry Wolf?

However, it is inarguable that bird flu is a potentially deadly illness. And the news media has been rife with stories theorizing that it could become the next great pandemic. Will bird flu kill hundreds of thousands, even millions, as some have predicted?

Simply put, no. It won't.

In November 2005, President George W. Bush wrote a letter to the public encouraging people to prepare "ourselves, our nation, and our world to fight this potentially devastating outbreak of infectious disease."[16]

But on April 14, 2006, Julie Gerberding, the head of the U.S. Centers for Disease Control and Prevention (CDC), participated in a conference designed to encourage state and local planning for pandemics, where she made statements that were in sharp contrast to those of President Bush.

In reference to the avian flu, Gerberding said that "there is no evidence that it will be the next pandemic."[17] She noted that although the disease has killed about half of the two hundred people known to have been infected with the virus, the victims were in intense, daily contact with sick flocks, often sharing the same living space, and that only two people had become infected by person-to-person contact.[18] She added that there was "no reason to think it ever will" pass easily between people.[19]

Gerberding urged the media to be cautious about how they report on the subject, and pointed out that "there will be temptation for the press to make this into something it is not." In order to prevent irrational panic, Gerberding called for "responsible journalism."[20]

> "There will be temptation for the press to make this into something it is not. We will need responsible journalism."
> —Julie Gerberding, head of the
> U.S. Centers for Disease Control and Prevention

Many others have attempted to make a similar point. Dr. Eva Wallner-Pendleton is an extension veterinarian and senior research associate at the Penn State Department of Veterinary and Biomedical Sciences. Her field of study includes diagnostic pathology of poultry, game birds, and exotic species. On April 18, 2006, Dr. Pendleton spoke about protecting small flocks from bird flu as part of a workshop on Avian Influenza (AI) and Current Poultry and Human Health Issues.[21] During her talk, she mentioned that she was actually more concerned about the spread of avian cholera on farms than she was about avian influenza.

She discouraged the audience from accepting the panic-driven "it's not if, it's when" approach to the bird flu issue. She urged public health officials and the media to take a more professional and measured response to the situation.

When a production crew from the Canadian Broadcasting Corporation (CBC) interviewed Vancouver's chief medical officer, Dr. John Blatherwick, they expected him to endorse the mainstream message of doom and gloom surrounding the bird flu pandemic.[22] Surprisingly, he laughed at the prospect: "You're more likely to be killing yourself eating big batches of fries and hamburgers—leading up to a heart attack—than you are to catch any of the diseases you're reading about . . . The avian flu is not going to be the next pandemic."[23]

Although Blatherwick agrees that preparedness is important in the event of a real emergency, he disparaged the "sky is falling" message and the idea of wasting resources on something that has yet to materialize. "Worry about walking across the street with the crazy drivers," he argued. "Worry about stuff that is real."[24]

Dr. Shiv Chopra, veterinarian and microbiologist, is just as critical of the idea that the H5N1 virus could cause a pandemic:

Infectious diseases in animals, including bird flu, can occasionally transmit to humans . . . But it does not then spread from a thus infected person to the next person to the next person. For example, people handling cattle or sheep carcasses can get anthrax but anthrax does not spread from people to people to cause human epidemics . . . Any microbiologist who tells you otherwise is lying. This is an absolute lie. It has not happened, it will not happen, it cannot happen. We know that from science."[25]

On May 22, 2006, the editors of *Maclean's* magazine wrote what seems to be a warning to the World Health Organization and other organizations involved in spreading fear about the bird flu. In their article "Paranoia, Bird Flu and the World Health Org," they wrote the following:

> . . . in recent years the World Health Organization has frequently allowed preparedness to mutate into paranoia. You'd think it would have learned from the SARS debacle, during which it issued a warning for foreign tourists to avoid Toronto, even though the outbreak was miniscule and quickly contained. Ebola and West Nile raised similar panics. When our guardians of global health tilt at every windmill on the epidemiological landscape they erode their own credibility. One day, there will be a genuine crisis. We can only hope that the public won't have tuned out the constant alarms.[26]

"Pandemic" Appears to Be Ending
Before It Even Began

In May 2006, Dr. David Nabarro, chief pandemic flu coordinator for the United Nations, announced that there have been fabulous success stories in Thailand and Vietnam concerning the H5N1 virus.[27]

Although health officials did not go so far as to say that H5N1 had been completely eradicated in those countries, they were pleased to note that in Vietnam, which has had almost half of the human cases of H5N1 flu in the world, they had not seen a single case in humans or a single outbreak in poultry all year.[28] Thailand, one of the hardest-hit nations behind Vietnam and Indonesia, had not had a human case in five months or one in poultry in six months.[29] They attributed their success to aggressive measures such as killing infected chickens, vaccinating healthy ones, protecting domestic flocks, and educating farmers.[30]

Also in May 2006, Wetlands International, one of the leading animal welfare agencies monitoring the bird flu, reported that birds migrating between Europe and Africa did not spread the virus that spring, as had been expected. Thousands of birds were tested, and not one case was found. Officials differ in their views, but many agree that it is highly unlikely that the H5N1 strain of the bird flu will arrive via migratory birds in North America. According to Ken Rosenberg, director of conservation science at the Cornell Lab of Ornithology, "If avian flu were to show up in U.S. poultry, migratory birds are probably the least likely source of infection."[31]

According to Maria Cheng, a spokeswoman for the World Health Organization, as of May 2006, "We haven't seen the virus move to as many countries as we saw in the beginning of the year."[32] Furthermore, she added, reports of human cases may be declining.[33] Even though the overall number of deaths had been declining, shortly after Cheng had made this remark several Indonesians died, raising the country's death toll to forty-one.

Human Infections from Bird Flu

One reason why the avian flu usually doesn't spread easily among humans is because it seems to infect cells deep in the lungs.[34] Theoretically, it is easier for a normal human flu strain to spread since it lives in the throat and nose, rather than deep in the lungs like the H5N1 virus. (It is thought that the normal flu virus is passed easily through sneezing.) Until recently, no evidence suggested that the highly infectious avian influenza virus was able to spread in the same manner as the normal flu.

In May 2006, seven Indonesians from the same family died from what appears to be the highly infectious avian flu. According to World Health Organization spokeswoman Maria Cheng, the first member of the Indonesian family to become sick was a thirty-seven-year-old woman who probably was infected while working at a market where there was poultry.[35] The woman fell ill in late April 2006 and died May 4.

Although it is believed that she died of bird flu, it has not been confirmed, because she was buried before anyone could take a test sample. Within two weeks of the woman's first symptoms, six family members who cared for her became sick. A seventh relative became sick about a week later. All of the infected family members tested positive for H5N1, and only one survived.

According to Cheng, over the last several years, there are at least three prior cases of the disease being circulated among family members. In September 2004, an eleven-year-old Thai girl infected her mother and her aunt after the two women spent hours at the girl's bedside caring for her. All three died. A similar cluster appeared earlier in Indonesia. Two family clusters in Vietnam also appear to fit a similar pattern.[36]

The eight-person case in Indonesia is considered the largest family cluster where the virus seems to have been transmitted from person to person since the H5N1 outbreak began in Hong Kong in 2003, according to World Health Organization spokesman Gregory Hartl.[37] So far, the family clusters show that only direct blood relatives—not spouses—have caught the bird flu. Hartl emphasizes that "human to human transmission can only occur when there is extensive and close contact between someone who is already show-ing clinical signs of the disease and the uninfected person."[38] Within the Indonesian family cluster in May/June 2006, the World Health Organization identified the first official case of human-to-human transfer of the H5N1 virus where a son passed on the disease to his father (again, they were in close proximity to each other).[39]

Indonesia has been criticized for not doing enough to prevent the spread of the bird flu, which has been found in twenty-seven out of thirty-three provinces.[40] The government admits that it cannot afford to destroy poultry, or pay to educate the peasants. Because animals roam wild through the villages, officials say that, in individual cases, they would have difficulty finding the possible "source" of the virus.

Many rural Indonesians also reject the idea that the bird flu is a problem and blame the deaths on "evil spirits." They don't trust government workers and are very suspicious of any efforts to test their animals. Millions in these countries rely on poultry as a principle food source and it only stands to reason that they would resist any efforts by the government to destroy their animals.

Since its first known attack on Indonesian poultry in late 2003, at least forty-one Indonesians have died of bird flu, the second high-est total in any country so far. As of June 6, 2006, a total of 225 cases of H5N1 avian influenza have been confirmed in Vietnam (93), Indonesia (53), Thailand (22), China (19), Egypt (14), Turkey (12), Azerbaijan (8), Cambodia (6), Iraq (2), and Djibouti (1), resulting in 132 deaths since December 2003.[41]

Remember, however, that most cases of avian influenza infec-tion in humans have resulted from direct or close contact with infected domestic poultry, or surfaces contaminated with secretions and excretions from infected birds, not from human-to-human transmission.[42] To date, there is little to no evidence to suggest that the H5N1 virus will lead to a pandemic.

Bird Flu Versus Seasonal Flu

Many of us have been inconvenienced by the common seasonal flu. For the average person, the flu is similar to a very bad cold. But influenza can also be more severe, and at times can lead to death. The elderly are considered to be more vulnerable, and according to the CDC, "deaths of older adults account for [more than] 90 percent of deaths attributed to pneumonia and influenza."[43]

The CDC currently says that the regular flu kills 36,000 people in the United States every year.[44] But some estimates indicate that through the 1970s and 1980s, there were 20,000 deaths per year from the flu. Now, suddenly, this figure has almost doubled. Why?

Harvard grad student Peter Doshi decided to do his own research into the claim that 36,000 people die annually from the flu. He published his letter "Are U.S. flu death figures more PR than science?" in the *British Medical Journal*.[45] He discovered that "between 1979 and 2002, the National Center for Health Statistics (NCHS) data show an average 1348 flu deaths per year (range 257 to 3006)."

If you're wondering why the CDC would inflate the number of flu deaths, keep in mind that the more people they can frighten into getting their flu shot, the greater profits for the vaccine manufacturers. If you believe the CDC's primary intention is to protect public health, you're wrong. Their goal seems more aligned with distorting disease data to convince more people that getting a flu shot makes sense. The CDC has an actual "recipe" for increasing flu shot demands.[46] The ingredients include:

- Concern

- Anxiety

- Fear

The fact is, government organizations like the CDC work hand in hand with businesses to sell products. I'll tell you more about why this is happening in later chapters.

In addition to the similarity between the symptoms of the bird flu and the seasonal flu, they are also both used by the marketing machines of the big drug companies to classically condition the population into believing that a vaccine is necessary to combat them both. Like Pavlov's dogs, people are "conditioned" into believing that a "shot" is the answer for these two "deadly" viruses. A great deal of marketing has gone into conditioning the masses into believing this.[47]

Tragically, a small number of the old and the frail do die of influenza every year—they can die from various causes. But does this justify all of us having to line up to get our vaccines? With so many other health crises occurring, why is the media so obsessed over this one particular health issue? Face it, if the story can't "sell" us something, there'd be no story.

Proper Perspective on Flu Deaths

To date, there have been no recorded cases of H5N1 in the United States And seasonal flu is a relatively minor problem in the United States compared to other illnesses. Each year, approximately 2.4 million Americans die from a variety of different causes. Yet many Americans have been led astray by the media hype. The headlines are preoccupying our minds with the bird flu pandemic at a completely disproportionate level.

According to the Centers for Disease Control and Prevention (CDC), 64,849 people died from pneumonia in 2000.[48] Furthermore, the CDC reports that more than 90 million Americans live with chronic illnesses that account for 70 percent of all deaths in the United States.[49] Seven of every ten Americans who die each year, or more than 1.7 million people, die of a chronic disease.[50]

CONDITIONS BY DEATHS[51]		
CONDITION	**U.S. DEATHS**	**DATA RESOURCE***
1. Death	2.4 million	1999 (NVHS Sep 2001)
2. Chronic Illness	1.6 million	(68.4% of deaths) from top 5 chronic diseases: heart disease, cancers, stroke, COPD, and diabetes (CDC/1999)
3. Cardiovascular diseases	945,836	(American Heart Association, 2004)
4. Heart disease	725,191	(NVSR Sep 2001); 30.3% of deaths
5. Cancer	555,500	(SEER 2002 estimate)
6. Ischemic heart disease	529,658	1999 (NVSR Sep 2001)
7. Coronary heart disease	502,188	2001 (American Heart Association, 2004)
8. Heart attack	459,841	1998 (NHLBI); 199,154 deaths for AMI reported in 1999 (NVSR Sep 2001)
9. Smoking	440,000	(CDC)
10. Obesity	300,000	(CDC)
11. Respiratory conditions	233,659	(NHLBI 1999)
12. Digestive diseases	191,000	1985 (Digestive diseases in the United States: Epidemiology and Impact—NIH Publication No. 94-1447, 1994)

Reproduced by permission from www.cureresearch.com

*NVHS (National Vital Health Statistics)
 CDC (Centers for Disease Control and Prevention)
 NVSR (National Vital Statistics Reports)
 NHLBI (National Heart, Lung and Blood Institute)
 NIH (National Institutes of Health)
 SEER (Surveillance, Epidemiology and End Results)

Throughout Asia, many of the rural poor simply don't even realize that there's a bird flu problem going on. Without media such as radios or televisions to tell them they should be afraid, they are more concerned with the diseases that are actually causing their deaths in large numbers, such as malaria, dysentery, and cholera.

Cholera is one of the most significant causes of illness and death in developing countries. It is caused by an intestinal infection that leads to very serious diarrhea, and it is still very prevalent in countries where overcrowding and poor sanitation are common. According to the World Health Organization, "Estimates of global cholera-specific mortality are believed to be 100,000 to 130,000 deaths per year, with most of the deaths occurring in Asia and Africa."[52] Tuberculosis kills nearly 2 million people every year, mostly in developing countries. Malaria causes more than 1 million deaths per year.[53]

According to Dr. William Legett Aldis, the WHO Representative in Thailand, "The South-East Asia Region alone counts for an estimated mortality of 800,000, representing about 40 percent of the global deaths due to diarrheal diseases, such as cholera and dysentery. Sadly enough, most of these occur in children under five years of age. Estimates of the environmental burden of disease revealed that, in developing countries, 85–90 percent of these deaths are attributable to the lack of safe water, sanitation and hygiene, i.e., an estimated total of about 700,000 deaths largely preventable if water and sanitation services were improved and basic rules of hygiene observed."[54]

He calls any efforts to provide developing countries with clean water a "collective failure" and believes millions of lives could be saved if sanitation were improved. According to Dr. Aldis, "Water sources [surface, underground and piped] are regularly subject to bacterial contamination with only about 50 percent of all supplies meeting the national drinking water standards."[55]

Learning from History

Plagues have killed millions of people worldwide since the dawn of civilization. It is difficult to determine the exact causes of many historic plagues. Some observations have been made, however, that implicate hygienic conditions and diet as being major contributing factors. For example, in 1665, the plague known as the Black Death arrived in London.[56] In the *Journal of the Plague Years*, author Daniel Defoe estimated that, in order to prevent the spread of the disease, 40,000 dogs and 200,000 cats were killed. As a result, there were fewer natural enemies of the rats who carried the plague fleas, so the germs spread more rapidly. As we will see later, Bill Dufty points out in his book, *Sugar Blues,* the poor diet also likely predisposed the Londoners to the illness by weakening their immune systems.

The current media hype emphasizes that if the bird flu virus mutates and becomes easily transmissible through human-to-human contact, it could kill millions of people worldwide. The rationale behind this prediction is based upon the outcome of other historical plagues before the implementation of acceptable hygiene and appropirate testing.

The theoretical bird flu pandemic is most frequently compared to the great Spanish flu outbreak of 1918, which afflicted millions of people worldwide. But in 1918, sanitation was nowhere near the levels we have today in the twenty-first century. The improvements in the safety of the U.S. water supply have greatly contributed to the reduction in the spread of disease. Also, the far superior communication systems available today enable us to respond quickly to almost any impending disaster.

The Spanish flu outbreak occurred during the legendarily harsh conditions of World War I, when thousands upon thousands of soldiers were packed together in filthy trenches. If you consider these factors, it becomes difficult to compare the circumstances of the Spanish flu, or any other historic plague, to current-day conditions in the North America. Rather than dwell on historic plague scenarios, it's more important to look at more current "plagues."

> The theoretical bird flu pandemic is most frequently compared to the great Spanish flu outbreak of 1918, which afflicted millions of people worldwide. But in 1918, sanitation was nowhere near the levels we have today in the twenty-first century.

If we fast-forward to 1976, we can examine the swine flu fiasco. We should all be reminded about the side effects of the swine flu vaccine campaign. Several hundred people developed crippling Guillain-Barré Syndrome after they were injected with this vaccine. Even healthy twenty-year-olds ended up as paraplegics in wheelchairs. Within a few months, claims totaling $1.3 billion had been filed by victims who had suffered paralysis from the swine flu vaccine. The vaccine was also blamed for twenty-five deaths. But the swine flu pandemic itself never materialized.[57]

The swine flu episode shows how difficult it is to forecast a pandemic and how damaging a rash response can be. More people died from the vaccine than died from the swine flu itself.

Investigative journalist Ida Honorof, credited by the *Los Angeles Times* and other publications with breaking some of the biggest stories of our time, called the political response to the swine flu panic "the most brazen, obscene electioneering ploy" ever, adding that it was proposed by the president "and his coterie of scientific hacks, fabricated to cause pure unadulterated panic and guarantee political capital, rammed through without consideration of people's health and lives and approved by a band-wagon Congress" eager to make the nation's "health" a bipartisan concern.[58]

In the case of the bird flu threat, it is important that history not repeat itself. The swine flu fiasco most likely could have been prevented had more people asked more questions. Hopefully, by asking enough questions about the bird flu, we can avoid the same devastating results.

Preparing for a pandemic is challenging, because it is difficult to strike a balance between acting and overreacting. President Bush and the rest of the world's leaders need to rise above panic and politics. They simply cannot afford to make the same mistake Gerald Ford made about the swine flu in 1976.

Unreasonable Measures to Control the "Pandemic"

Other than washing your hands more often or wearing face masks, another proposed method to control the spread of a pandemic is to quarantine affected areas. Historically, one of the main public health techniques has been to quarantine sections of the human population.

In May 2006, after a dead chicken was discovered to have been infected with the H5N1, quarantines were imposed in some communities in Romania. Romania had previously experienced other bird flu outbreaks in 2005, without a human death. But after the single dead chicken was found, several thousand people were quarantined as a preventative measure, despite the fact that not one person had contracted the flu.

Initially, the quarantine was to last three weeks. Police were patrolling the streets, houses were disinfected, chickens were culled, and drugs were handed out at no charge. Many Romanians were noncompliant and angry about the quarantine and accused government officials of overreacting. The populace was completely un-prepared for a quarantine, and many found themselves without food or water and were forced to leave their homes in search of sup-plies. Many mocked the idea that a sick bird could warrant the measures being taken, and the quarantines were quickly lifted as a result of the protests against them. In the end, the quarantine only lasted four days.[59]

As a measure to control the spread of the highly pathogenic bird flu, H5N1, some countries have imposed bans at certain times and in specified locations on outdoor poultry, including Austria, Canada, China, Croatia, France, Germany, Italy, The Netherlands, Nigeria, Norway, Slovenia, Sweden, Switzerland, Thailand, Ukraine, and Vietnam.[60] Although many of these bans have been lifted, the ban in Quebec, Canada, which began on November 12, 2005, is still being imposed. Ironically, this ban was passed even though there has been no incidence of H5N1 in Canada. A group of farmers in Quebec, Union Paysanne, believe that the ban is based on un-founded science and is currently working on getting it lifted.[61] Forced confinement threatens the livelihoods of small pastured poultry producers who raise their chickens outdoors.

So far, officials have tried to push the envelope to see just how people will react. It's clear that whether officials try to destroy or confine poultry or even quarantine humans, there could be much resistance.

Selling a Pandemic

With television ads and newscasters telling us to get ready for a deadly pandemic, many people are now conveniently primed to take drugs such as Tamiflu or line up to be injected with a vaccine. Because of the media, people are being conditioned to think that the only solution comes from the government or the corporations.

Although it's true that it's important to be prepared for any disaster, there are many things you can do to prevent disease. For one, you can seek out healthier sources of chicken from local pastured poultry operations. Making other healthy diet and lifestyle choices will help boost your immune systems so that you minimize your chances of getting sick. If your only sources of information are the television, radio, and newspapers, you probably haven't been informed of these other choices.

But other choices do exist—they simply aren't choices that increase corporate profits or lead to exciting news stories. The public seems to crave the excitement that comes with being frightened, and reporters happily oblige, as it helps sell more newspapers and magazines, retains a radio audience, and keeps the viewers watching TV. And, as you will learn in the next chapter, that makes the media's corporate sponsors very happy indeed.

Recent Tracking of the H5N1 Bird Flu[62, 63, 64]

1996—Virus is found in a farmed goose in Guangdong province, southern China.

1997—Six deaths, eighteen people hospitalized. To control the outbreak, 1.5 million chickens are killed. Outbreaks of the virus are reported in poultry at farms and wet markets in Hong Kong.

February 2003—Two cases of the virus (one fatal) are confirmed in a Hong Kong family with a recent travel history to Fujian Province, China. A third family member dies of severe respiratory disease while in mainland China, but no samples are taken.

Wave I

December 2003—Two tigers and two leopards, fed fresh chicken carcasses, die unexpectedly at a zoo in Thailand. This is the first report of influenza causing disease and death in big cats.

December 2003—Republic of Korea confirms virus as cause of poultry deaths at three farms.

January 2004—Thailand and Vietnam report human and poultry cases.

January 2004—Japan, Cambodia, and Lao PDR report virus in poultry.

February 2004—In Thailand, scientists confirm that the disease has killed fourteen of fifteen housecats kept by one family who had seen one of the cats scavenging a dead chicken. All of the cats fell ill, but one recovered.

February 2004—Virus reported in poultry in Indonesia and China.

March 2004—In total, twelve cases (eight fatal) occur in Thailand and twenty-three cases (sixteen fatal) occur in Vietnam.

Wave II

June–July 2004—China, Indonesia, Thailand, and Vietnam report recurrence of virus in poultry.

August–September 2004—Vietnam reports four new human cases, all fatal. Malaysia reports H5N1 in poultry.

September–October 2004—Thailand reports five cases, four fatal. Outbreak begins in zoo tigers in Thailand said to have been fed chicken carcasses. Altogether, 147 tigers out of 441 die or are euthanized. H5N1 is confirmed in two eagles illegally imported into Brussels from Thailand.

November 2004—Five cases (four fatal) occur in Thailand and four cases, all fatal, occur in Vietnam.

Wave III

December 2004—Poultry outbreaks ongoing in Indonesia, Thailand, and Vietnam and possibly also in Cambodia and Lao PDR. Vietnam reports new human case.

January 2005—Vietnam reports two further human cases. Total cases in Vietnam rise to six. Sporadic cases continue to be reported over the coming months, making Vietnam the hardest-hit country.

February–May 2005—Cambodia reports four human cases, which are fatal.

February 2005—H5N1—Vietnam reports thirteen new infections, twelve deaths.

February–May 2005—H5N1—Cambodia reports first case, second, third, and fourth cases, all fatal.

April 2005—H5N1—Wild birds begin dying at Qinghai Lake in central China, where hundreds of thousands of migratory birds congregate. Altogether, 6,345 birds from different species die in the coming weeks.

June 2005—H5N1—China reports poultry outbreak in Xinjiang Autonomous Region.

July 2005—H5N1—Indonesia reports their first human case. Infection in two other family members is considered likely but cannot be confirmed.

July 2005—H5N1—Russia reports outbreaks in poultry in western Siberia. The outbreak spreads to affect six administrative regions in Siberia. Dead migratory birds are reported in the vicinity of outbreak.

August 2005—H5N1—Kazakhstan reports an outbreak of the virus in poultry in areas adjacent to Siberia. Dead migratory birds are reported in the vicinity of the outbreaks.

August 2005—Since November 2004, Vietnam now has sixty-four confirmed cases, of which twenty-one were fatal.

August 2005—China reports outbreak in birds in Tibet Autonomous Region. Mongolia reports the death of eighty-nine migratory birds at two lakes.

October 2005—Taiwan and China report the detection of virus in a cargo of exotic songbirds smuggled from mainland China. Virus is also confirmed in an imported parrot, held in quarantine in the UK, that died three days earlier.

October 2005—China reports outbreak in birds in Hunan, making this the sixth province reporting outbreaks during 2005.

September–October 2005—Indonesia confirms second, third, fourth, and fifth cases.

October 2005—Virus confirmed in poultry in Turkey and Romania. Croatia confirms virus in wild birds. New human case confirmed in Thailand (first since October 2004). Thailand and Indonesia report more human cases.

November 2005—Vietnam reports its first new human case since July 2005. China reports its third human case and more outbreaks in poultry. Sporadic human cases to be reported in the coming weeks.

December 2005—Ukraine reports its first outbreak in domestic birds. Turkey reports outbreak in birds. Kuwait detects first case of virus in a single migratory flamingo.

January 2006—Turkey reports its first two human cases and outbreaks in poultry. Sporadic human cases continue to be reported in the coming weeks. Iraq reports its first human case.

February–March 2006—H5N1—These are the most active months in H5N1 history:

- Nigeria reports first H5N1 cases in chickens. Five farms are infected.

- Iraq reports outbreak in backyard flocks in same province where human case detected. Iraq reports a second human death within thirteen new cases.

- Indonesia reports its twenty-fifth case and eighteenth fatality.

- China reports its twelfth case and eighth fatality.

- Malaysia confirms virus in a flock of free-range poultry.

- Greece, Italy, Germany, Iran, Austria, Slovenia, Slovakia, Bosnia-Herzegovina, Georgia, Serbia-Montenegro, Hungary, Poland, Czech Republic, and Bulgaria report swans infected with H5N1.

- Albania confirms virus in poultry (chickens).

- Azerbaijan reports H5N1-infected dead birds floating in the Caspian Sea and reports first human cases.

- European countries begin ordering all domestic birds be kept indoors, including zoos.

- Egypt reports virus in domestic poultry and confirms its first human case.

- Sweden reports infection in wild birds (ducks) and in a mink.

- France confirms virus in a wild duck.

- India reports eight human H5N1 cases and confirms virus in domestic poultry.

- Spain reports H5N1-infected dead duck.

- Italy reports sixteen new H5N1 cases.

- India confirms virus in domestic poultry and orders the slaughter of 500,000 chickens.

- Russia reports the first outbreaks at large commercial farms.

- Denmark reports thirty-five H5N1-infected dead birds.

- To date, 200 million chickens have been slaughtered.

- France reports H5N1 bird flu in thousands of dead commercial turkeys and one dead wild duck.

- Switzerland reports first H5N1 case in a duck.

- Denmark confirms virus in a wild bird.

- Niger reports H5N1-infected dead ducks—bare hands, no face masks on disposal team.

- Austria and Germany reports dead cats infected with H5N1.

- Israel confirms virus in poultry.

- Germany confirms virus in a stone marten.

- Cameroon confirms virus in domestic duck.

- Myanmar, Jordan, and Pakistan confirm virus in poultry.

- Cambodia confirms its first human case since April 2005.

April–May 2006

- Egyptian girl dies of H5N1 infection.

- Burkina Faso, Sudan, Côte d'Ivoire, and Germany confirm virus in poultry.

- A fourth Afghan province, Kapisa, is hit; poultry is culled and quarantine measures are introduced in affected areas.

- To date, there is only one confirmed case of H5N1 in the UK—in a dead wild bird (swan).

- Seven family members dead due to H5N1 infection in Indonesia.

2

SENSATION SELLS

How and Why the Media Deceives You about the Bird Flu

"Media is still the best way to learn about the world, and one way to change it. Technology alone is not a solution. More of a commitment to democracy by the media could be. And that means you!"[1]

—DANNY SCHECHTER,
director of *WMD: Weapons of Mass Deception*

Most of us are oblivious to the tactics that are regularly used to deceive us into submission. But you have the power to reject the fraudulent and manipulative tactics used by the media to control you, once you become aware of what they are. The media has the ability to influence and manipulate your thoughts, preventing you from thinking for yourself.

Those who wish to exploit your senses in order to manipulate you into believing their promises and accepting without question their pitches have mastered the art of using fear to fool you into believing their false promises. According to media analyst Nelson Thall, the former Chief Archivist for the McLuhan Center on Global Communications, "They create the disease in order to offer the cure. For those in control, the 'disease' is to instill fear among the masses. For them, the 'cure' is to get the people to give up their freedoms, liberties, rights and identities. That's how those in control think." When asked if he thought the bird flu would exist without the help of the media, Thall responded, "The BIRD FLU—emphasis—wouldn't exist without the help of the media. The bird flu, yes. But, not the BIRD FLU!"[2]

You are being tricked into believing that the media is telling you the truth and that only Big Pharma has the answers to your health problems.

> "To the future or to the past, to a time when thought is free, when men are different from one another and do not live alone—to a time when truth exists and what is done cannot be undone: From the age of uniformity, from the age of solitude, from the age of BIG BROTHER, from the age of doublethink—greetings!"
>
> —GEORGE ORWELL, *1984* [3]

Desire for the Latest Is a Dual-Edged Sword

New inventions make us all feel better. We yearn for the newest, biggest HDTV, the fanciest cell phones, the latest games stations, the fastest computers, and the smallest and best iPod. When the latest gadget is released on the market, consumers race to be the first to buy one. When something is new and "upgraded," the associated excitement tends to grab our attention.

On the other hand, when something is old, repetitive, or redundant, we frequently become disinterested and bored. Most of us strive to improve ourselves, and when we do, we feel a great sense of accomplishment. The one-upmanship that is associated with new technologies makes us feel as though, somehow, society is making progress.

Like new technologies, news stories must always be new and exciting to the viewing audience; otherwise, they'll switch to another channel. The networks know this, and in order to improve or maintain viewers, they milk stories like the bird flu for all they're worth. Bird flu is a new "story" that will scare the people and bring them into their programming. People have become bored hearing about cancer and heart disease, so why not stir up the pot with the dreaded "bird flu"?

> News stories must always be new and exciting to the viewing audience; otherwise, they'll switch to another channel. The networks know this, and in order to improve or maintain viewers, they milk stories like the bird flu for all they're worth.

The constant desire for new technologies may have an upside as well. Millions of Web sites, blogs, and chat rooms are available on the Internet that allow those who do know enough to ask more questions to search for alternative viewpoints on a variety of subjects. For those who have been in control of the media, the shift of viewers from the television to the Internet could adversely affect their revenue streams. The Internet is an attractive option for news seekers, as it offers the first real hope of finding information that is truly independent and not influenced by corporate interests. However, the Internet has been both a blessing and a curse, confusing people as much as it has also been informing them.

Home Broadband Penetration[4]
(% of all adult Americans with high speed at home)

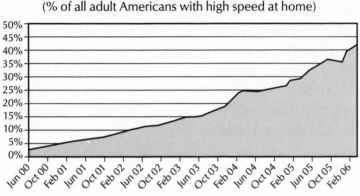

John B. Horrigan, Home Broadband Adoption 2006, Pew Internet & American Life Project, May 28, 2006
http://www.pewinternet.org/pdfs/PIP_Broadband_trends2006.pdf

Percentage of U.S. Adults Online[5]

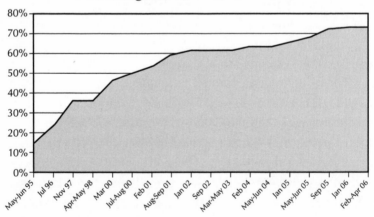

Pew Internet & American Life Project Surveys, March 2000–April 2006
http://www.pewinternet.org/trends/Internet_Adoption_4.26.06.pdf

According to a study by Pew Internet and American Life Project Surveys, 84 million Americans currently have broadband at home, and 73 percent of U.S. adults used the Internet in 2006, up from 60 million and 66 percent in 2005.[6] The most frequently viewed online video category is the news.[7] Fifty million Americans turn to the Internet for news on a typical day.[8]

This may be hard to imagine now, but one day, the television may become an antiquated technology. Television is bound to gradually lose its audience to the Internet, where people are able to find independent news and views that can inform, rather than propagandize. Additionally, Web 2.0 technologies will allow them to interactively participate with the news process, and actually participate in choosing newsworthy stories, as is already being done on Web sites like Digg.com.

On the Internet, people have the opportunity to seek out unbiased news—news that simply would never be told in the mainstream media. As people seek out free-flowing information on the Internet, those in control of mainstream media may eventually hit a brick wall. It may only be a matter of time before the masses realize just how much censorship exists in the corporately controlled media. It's possible that people will someday look back at these tactics and laugh, seeing the strategy for what it was—sophisticated psychological mind-control programming.

> "Media concentration is a dagger in America's heart—the First Amendment . . . The only Americans with meaningful First Amendment rights today are those who own the media . . . Unless you have billions in spare pocket change and buy one of the Big Ten [media corporations] for yourself, you're out of the game. Silenced."
>
> —NICHOLAS JOHNSON,
> FCC commissioner from 1966 to 1973[9]

Propaganda and Mind Control

Edward L. Bernays, author of the book *Propaganda*, is considered to be the "Father of Spin." He mastered the art of persuading the masses using ideas he learned from his uncle, Sigmund Freud. As a marketing genius, he could convince anybody to buy just about anything. He described the public as a "herd that needed to be led." His public relations campaigns were so smooth in their approach that the public was unaware that they were even being manipulated. He believed that the public needed to be told what to think because they were incapable of creating their own rational thought.

In *Propaganda*, Bernays writes:

> Those who manipulate the unseen mechanism of society constitute an invisible government which is the true ruling power of our country. We are governed, our minds molded, our tastes formed, our ideas suggested largely by men we have never heard of. This is a logical result of the way in which our democratic society is organized. Vast numbers of human beings must cooperate in this manner if they are to live together as a smoothly functioning society. In almost every act of our lives, whether in the sphere of politics or business in our social conduct or our ethical thinking, we are dominated by the relatively small number of persons who understand the mental processes and social patterns of the masses. It is they who pull the wires that control the public mind.[10]

Whether you read a newspaper, listen to the radio, watch television, or surf the Internet, you run the risk of being manipulated and deceived by this type of propaganda. On the other hand, if you're careful, you can learn the truth. The trick to being able to differentiate between reality and the lies and deception may be as simple as learning to follow the money trail.

Once you learn how to follow the money, piercing the veil of deception will become much easier for you. When you follow the money, you can frequently uncover and understand hidden agendas and conflicts of interest. Suddenly, the common strategies that many corporations use to deceive you become clearly transparent. You won't need to rely on any "experts" to help you sort through the confusion, as you will be able to see right through many of the disinformation schemes yourself.

Since the dawn of civilization, propaganda has been used to manipulate belief systems. Ultimately, it is the responsibility of each individual to properly interpret the goal of the messages being spread through any given medium.

Fatal Contact—An Example of How Media Was Used to Distort Reality About the Bird Flu

On May 9, 2006, ABC aired the movie *Fatal Contact: Bird Flu in America*. The introduction to the movie included a type of "disclaimer," labeling the movie as a "fictional examination" about what would happen "if" there were a bird flu pandemic. There was a similar type of disclaimer at the end of the movie.

Rampant throughout the movie were scenes of people desperate for a cure, and demanding to know why the government didn't prepare for the pandemic by developing a vaccine. If the network's goal was to help stimulate a demand for H5N1 vaccine, then the movie may have been a success.

The movie aired on May 9, just four days after President Bush had announced that he was allocating $1 billion to five companies to develop vaccines against seasonal influenza or a pandemic strain. After seeing the film, many probably were relieved that the announcement had been made. It's an incredibly brilliant form of marketing—to paint a disaster in a fictional setting in order to create a receptive mind-set for vaccines and drugs as a possible solution.

> It's an incredibly brilliant form of marketing—to paint a disaster in a fictional setting in order to create a receptive mind-set for vaccines and drugs as a possible solution.

I suspect GlaxoSmithKline, MedImmune Inc., Novartis AG, Computer Sciences Corp unit DynPort Vaccine Co, Baxter International Inc., and Solvay Pharmaceuticals considered the movie worthy of a five-star rating.

Companies Benefiting from the Billion-Dollar Windfall:[11]

GlaxoSmithKline PLC	$274.75 million
MedImmune Inc.	$169.46 million
Novartis AG	$220.51 million
Computer Sciences Corp (Dynport Vaccine Corp working with Baxter International Inc.)	40.97 million
Solvay Pharmaceuticals	$298.59 million

In Raleigh, North Carolina, the ABC affiliate posted a phone number at the bottom of the screen for people to call if they had any questions for the local state health department concerning the bird flu. A similar system was set in place in Pittsburgh, Pennsylvania. Both the Raleigh and Pittsburgh public health departments fielded hundreds of calls after the movie aired.

In order to point out the impact the movie had on the viewers, here is a sample of some of the questions asked to Dr. Leah Devlin at the North Carolina Department of Human Health Services:

- Why are people getting flu shots? Is this something that everyone should be doing? Can the flu shot prevent people from getting sick with the bird flu?

- When is the H5N1 virus expected to hit?

- Is the bird flu here in the States already?

- Are the surgical masks that people are wearing in the movie effective in preventing transmission, or are stronger N95 masks required?

- How likely are people to die from the bird flu if they do contract it?

- Is the Tamiflu vaccine available now? Do all birds have the potential to carry the bird flu?

- Will the bird flu be a health issue that we will have to worry about for years to come?

- In the movie, the quarantine was not working. Do you feel a quarantine will be effective? And how will this work?

- Are there statewide plans to secure neighborhoods in the event of an outbreak?

The movie was supposedly "entertainment" and was not described as a documentary. But the call-in numbers make it clear that, despite the disclaimers, the viewers were being encouraged to look at the movie as being serious and factual. For all intents and purposes, the movie was as much a commercial for the bird flu "industry" as it was "entertainment."

Fatal Contact: Bird Flu in America didn't do very well in the ratings, averaging a paltry 5.3 million viewers. *American Idol* led the night with 28.1 million viewers.[12] But 5.3 million viewers still adds up to a lot of potential vaccine customers.

On March 6, 2006, two months before the movie aired, a poll conducted by the *Washington Post* revealed that 60 percent of Americans are concerned about avian influenza, but fewer than 34 percent think it will appear in the United States this year.[13]

This is bad news for people who stand to gain from "stirring the pot." Nothing would please them more than having more people think that the bird flu will hit the United States by the end of the year, because those who believe that the avian flu will be a problem will be the first in line for a vaccine. *Fatal Contact* is just one part of a wide media propaganda assault designed to increase that number.

The United States Is One of the Few Countries in the World Where Drug Companies Are Allowed to Advertise Prescription Drugs Directly to Consumers

Even a cursory review of TV commercials will help you understand the powerful connection between the pharmaceutical companies and the networks. Without the sponsorship money coming in from multinational drug corporations, the networks wouldn't have grown to be as powerful as they are today. Likewise for Big Pharma—without the networks, drug companies would have a significantly smaller market share. With so much money coming in from the drug companies, it only stands to reason that the networks would do everything in their power to cooperate with just about any agenda Big Pharma wanted to promote.

According to Dr. Mary Beth Pinto, "Pharmaceutical companies spent $40 million on media advertising for direct-to-consumer prescription drugs in 1989. By 1995, this amount has risen to $350 million, for the first time matching the industry's spending on advertising to physicians and other professionals. Total direct-to-consumer advertising revenues have recently topped $1.5 billion."[14]

One way to minimize the influence of the drug companies through the media networks would be to reenact the ban on direct-to-consumer commercials that existed prior to 1997. The United States and New Zealand are the only two countries in the world that allow drug companies to advertise directly to consumers.[13]

If this ban could ever be reenacted, then scare campaigns such as the avian flu would be much harder to successfully pull off. News stories about the avian flu are not news; they are ads used to manipulate viewers to want either Tamiflu or the bird flu vaccine.

Sixty-six percent of U.S. media professionals say financial bottom-line pressure is "seriously hurting" the quality of news coverage.[16a]

Fifty-six percent of the U.S. population feel media reports are inaccurate.[16b]

Seventy percent believe that news organizations are "often influenced by powerful people and corporations."[16c]

Scaring You Is Nothing New

The story of the "bird flu" scare is not new. We've seen similar calls to alarm repeatedly throughout history, but they have been magnified over the last several decades with the help of ever more sophisticated forms of media manipulation. The incessant barrage of other panics we've been subjected to seems to have "normalized" fear into our culture. Without fear we'd buy less, and we'd also probably have less to talk about.

Think of the swine flu, Ebola, the West Nile virus, SARS, anthrax, or mad cow disease. Do they make the bird flu alarm seem more familiar? Think about the "preparing for the worst" messages from the media in the lead-up to Y2K. The media used intense and clever techniques to lure their viewers into believing that these stories were true, and that these dangers were likely to manifest. The networks are becoming more and more aggressive in seeking to convince you that what they are showing is, in fact, "reality."

Why do they want to frighten you? For one thing, if you're scared, you'll keep watching to find out more, and they can maintain their ratings and sell ads to tempt you with even more goods. Failure to accomplish this goal would mean a reduction of revenue from their sponsors.

Additionally, people who are frightened buy more. They stockpile against disaster, demand vaccines, buy expensive devices to keep themselves safe or make themselves feel better. That also makes the sponsors very happy.

> **"Covering the news, once seen primarily as a public service that could also make a profit, became primarily a vehicle for attracting audiences and selling advertising to make money."**
>
> —LEONARD DOWNIE JR. and ROBERT KAISER,
> *The News About the News: American Journalism in Peril*[17]

Now, I was trained as a Boy Scout and firmly believe in the motto of being prepared. Having disaster-contingency supplies in your home makes perfect sense. Having a supply of food, water, and portable power is a great form of insurance for a variety of natural disasters, not just the bird flu. But many people are scared out of all proportion to the actual dangers, while remaining uninformed about much more real and present dangers that the media and their sponsors ignore.

Today, we have been manipulated away from an accurate understanding of health, and many of us are now pursuing lifestyles that allow chronic disease and suffering to become the norm, rather than the rare exception. Hearing about healthy eating and locally grown foods is just simply not very exciting. If Hollywood or the networks did a movie about this, it would likely be a major flop.

So the media is focused on presenting a fear-based scenario that predisposes you to surrender your money to their sponsors. It's just that simple.

> **"I think the idea of creating a television news source that is not beholden to corporate interests is nirvana. It's apparently the only chance we're going to have to feature news reporters who are willing to behave inelegantly by sticking their nose under the tent to learn what the righteous and powerful have in store for us."**
>
> —PHIL DONAHUE[18]

One particularly disturbing result of this culture of fear is that it also allows the government to take away more and more of your freedoms. In May 2006, *USA Today* revealed that the National Security Association (NSA) has been secretly collecting the phone-call records of tens of millions of Americans, using data freely submitted to them by the phone companies.[19]

The phone companies are currently claiming that they did not provide this information. But whether or not this collection of data actually occurred, public opinion regarding the issue was disturbingly positive. Previously such an abrogation of our privacy would have caused a major outrage. But the following day the *Washington Post* reported that 63 percent of Americans were actually in favor of this collection.[20] Why? Because they justified this invasion of privacy as an acceptable way to combat terrorism.

In a similar way, the culture of fear can be used by large corporations to push passage of legislation that is favorable to them. You'll read later about how fear of mad cow disease has led to the proposed National Animal Identification System (NAIS), which could drive many small farmers out of business.

Who's Responsible for the Decline in Health in the United states?

With the bird flu scare, doctors are now seeing patients obsessing over the possibility of contracting the bird flu. People have been blindsided by the media hype and are overlooking many other important health issues. While they demand vaccines for a pandemic that will never come, they have never been told about the real health problems and solutions that could truly affect their lives.

While the corporations increase their stranglehold on every media outlet and you are bombarded with stories about theoretical "plagues," some very real epidemics are going on with almost no reporting at all. Two-thirds of Americans are overweight, 73 million have diabetes or prediabetes,[21, 22] and 8 million will come down with Alzheimer's by 2030 in the United States.[23] More than 1,300,000 new cancer cases and nearly 600,000 cancer deaths were expected in the United States in 2005,[24] and in early 2005 it was announced that cancer passed heart disease as the top killer of Americans.[25] Clearly, the conventional system of providing health news has not been effective at halting the progress of chronic degenerative diseases in the United States.

With all of this news about health and nearly daily breakthroughs in medicine, why are so many people still suffering? And why does the United States pay more than $2 trillion dollars a year for health care, more than any other country in the world, and yet rank only forty-eighth in the world in life expectancy?[26] Something is desperately wrong with this picture.

One contributing factor to the decline in the quality of our health has to do with the deterioration in the quality of our food. Since the beginning of the last century, our food supply has changed dramatically, to processed, prepackaged food created and distributed primarily by large corporations. As our food supply has changed, our health has correspondingly deteriorated.

You may wonder just how the corporations have been able to get away with selling you substandard food. It's one thing for the media to "sell" these foods with their ads, but what about the supposedly authoritative reports we hear about the modern diet, and the science that is behind them? We're often told that "experts agree" and that "experts support" and that "experts declare" some new health insight regarding food or nutrition. What the viewers should be asking themselves, though, is who funded the research that allows these "experts" to make these claims, and do these "experts" have any financial ties to the products they are promoting? Maybe if we asked more questions about oour food and nutrition, we wouldn't see the health or crisis we have today.

If you want to find the truth, it's important to follow the money. Unfortunately, the sad reality is that there frequently is very little money to be made in telling you the truth.

Corruption in Science Is Far More Common than You May Think

If the public would delve more deeply into the agendas behind stories like the bird flu, they would find many scientific holes in the positions being taken. For instance, as you will see later, science does not support the theory that the highly pathogenic bird flu virus can spread through human-to-human transmission. Certain interests benefit by spreading this theory and claiming that it is based on truthful science, when it is not.

Unfortunately, it seems clear that many scientific endeavors have become progressively more corrupted with funding conflicts of interest. We've always been exposed to corruption, but over the course of the last century, corruption in the sciences has gone from bad to worse. Honest, unbiased, objective science should be commended. But what about science that isn't so honest? What is done when a scientist lies in order to please the corporation or university he or she is working for? Don't forget that many universities are financially dependent upon corporate grant money.

According to Ghislaine Lanctôt, a former medical doctor and author of the book *Medical Mafia*, when you don't follow what Big Money wants, you get what she calls the "sticks":

> Sticks are used to beat you up for not following the herd. Disobedient people are the ones who don't serve big money. The first stick is the "stick of exclusion." You'll be fired. That stops 95 percent of the people from speaking up.
>
> The second stick is the "stick of dispossession." You'll have your title taken away. You'll have your right of titles taken away. You'll have your prestige taken away. You'll be put down. Your money will be taken away. Your house, your car . . . anything that will make you shut up.
>
> If that is not enough, then the third stick is the "stick of elimination." You'll be put in jail or a mental institution. . . . The question is, "Are we going to be afraid of the sticks?"[27]

Paul Connett, PhD is a specialist in Environmental Chemistry and Toxicology, and professor of chemistry at St. Lawrence University. He is also very concerned about the state of science today. In his words:

If public health policy is not supported by honest science, then we're in deep, deep trouble. Not only because we're not getting the right public policy, but because there will be a complete lack of trust when people find out the truth. We need to trust these agencies (CDC, NIH, etc.). If the CDC tells us we need to worry about something, we may completely ignore them because we've become so immune to their lies . . . We need to cut the cancer of dishonest science out of public health policy.[28]

Corporations have funneled a great deal of money into universities, and as a result, the universities have been more than happy to produce scientific data that suits the corporations' needs. Jennifer Washburn, a freelance journalist who is concerned about the influence that corporations have over our universities, says in her book *University Inc: The Corporate Corruption of Higher Education*:

Corporate funding of universities is growing and the money comes with strings attached. In return for this largesse, universities are acting more and more like for-profit patent factories, while professors are behaving more like businessmen. Secrecy is replacing the free flow of basic knowledge, university funds are shifting from the humanities to more commercially lucrative science labs, and the skill of teaching is valued less and less.[29]

Paul Connett, already quoted above, is likewise appalled by the corruption in science going on at the universities:

One of the worst offenders on that is Harvard. With the Harvard name on the top of your paper you can literally get away with murder . . . a number of prestigious scientists at Harvard have whitewashed toxics for industry. There is a lot of evidence that shows that when industry funds studies, the results go in one way and when it's not industry funded the results go in a different way. There is a very clear relationship between who's funding the study and the outcome you get.[30]

Lobbying Is Big Business

Even when legitimate science is able to escape unscathed from the corporate funding system and rampant conflicts of interest, regulations and laws are often still based on the desires of big business rather than any kind of sound science. Since 2000, the number of registered lobbyists in Washington DC has more than doubled.[31,32] In 2004, lobbyists generated a whopping $2.1 billion, with food and agricultural lobbying accounting for at least $51 million. Also in 2004, agribusiness companies contributed an additional $52.7 million to political campaigns.[33]

As Anna Lappé and Bryant Terry point out in their book *Grub*, this means that "beyond their budgets for advertising, public relations, and other media, the food industry and their employees spent at least $105 million on political influence during just one year."[34]

Lobbyists are hired by many different industries to influence decisions made by the government. And they are very successful at doing just that. A report prepared by Rep. Henry A. Waxman, "Politics and Science in the Bush Administration," says the following:

> The American people depend upon federal agencies to promote scientific research and to develop science-based policies that protect the nation's health and welfare . . . Recently, however, leading scientific journals have begun to question whether scientific integrity at federal agencies has been sacrificed to further a political and ideological agenda.[35]

The report finds numerous instances of the scientific process being distorted, or scientific findings being suppressed.

Luise Light, M.S. Ed.D., former USDA director of dietary guidance and nutrition education research, was responsible for creating the original food pyramid and revamping the USDA's nutrition information. In her book *What to Eat: The Ten Things You Really Need to Know to Eat Well and Be Healthy*, she exposes stories of corruption she witnessed while she was working at the USDA. She also tells the real story behind what happened to the food pyramid.

Here is just one of her stories:

> The original food pyramid I was in charge of developing was not allowed to be published, and a series of bright new, updated publications about diet and health were "deep-sixed," never to be distributed by USDA again because they didn't follow the new party line: that all food is good food . . . Those of us who were trying to offer the public the truth about food, nutrition, and health, which was our job, were quickly sidetracked . . .
>
> In my case, I was taken to the posh hotel . . . for a meeting . . . At that meeting, I was offered an attaché case full of money (sixty thousand dollars) for eliminating all mention of the word cancer in a new nutrition and health program I was developing for the American Red Cross.[36]

She didn't take the bribe.

With so much corruption surrounding the relationship between government, science, and the food industry, it's no surprise that the quality of our food supply has significantly deteriorated. According to the Centers for Disease Control and Prevention (CDC), there are more than 250 foodborne diseases.[37] The CDC estimates that in the United States alone, food poisoning causes about 76 million illnesses, 325,000 hospitalizations, and up to 5,000 deaths each year.[38]

When you consider the numbers associated with food poisoning, you would think that the government would be concerned about creating better regulations for our food supply. When you add in threats such as the bird flu, genetically modified foods, perchlorate, pesticides, acrylamide, trans fats, MSG, artificial sweeteners, and many other substances in our food that could compromise our health, the need for good regulation becomes critical. Instead, however, efforts are underway to deregulate our food supply.

Dr. Luise Light is appalled by a current bill (4167) designed to deregulate the food supply:

> In a diabolical move to eliminate three out of every four U.S.
> food-safety regulations with a single stroke of the pen, the food
> industry has written and handed off to this Congress a bill that
> would make federal agencies such as FDA, EPA, and USDA the
> only ones who can develop and enforce food-safety rules to pro-
> tect the public. It cancels out the traditional role of the states,
> which have been more aggressive and quicker to act to protect
> people from dangers in their food. Why is that? The federal agen-
> cies have been in bed with the agribusiness, food, and drug
> industries for decades![39]

Do Not Always Trust Foundations

The next time you hear a news story about an issue such as the bird flu, take a step back and realize that some very sophisticated and organized propaganda and corporate media relations went into the development of that story. Stories about the bird flu are not provided to help you; their intention is to scare you into buying something.

Valid and uncompromised research studies that are able to navigate their way through the universities, government, and corporate pressure still must face yet another line of defense from big business:

"independent" groups created by corporations to promote highly inaccurate pseudo-science in order to counter the real data. The corporations have not only exploited the media, government, and universities to support the sales of their products, they have also enrolled the help of "front groups" or innocent-sounding "foundations" to act in their favor.

Edward Bernays, author of *Propaganda*, knew that the most effective way to manipulate people into buying a product is through "independent third-party" endorsements.[40] Many of these "independent third-party" experts have come up with strategies to convince people that it's perfectly all right to be exposed to dangerous drugs, vaccines, pesticides, perchlorate, MSG, aspartame, acrylamide, benzene, and other toxins.

According to John Stauber, coauthor of *Trust Us, We're Experts!*, "Powerful corporate interests have learned to hide behind front groups with noble sounding names such as the American Council on Science and Health, the Harvard Center for Risk Analysis and the Center for Consumer Freedom."[41]

Bernays himself established several foundations that served to clean up the images of certain corporations in order to make consumers feel more comfortable with them. These foundations were designed to put out scientific studies and press materials that suited the needs of the corporations.

These types of foundations deliver the impression that they are working for you; however, their actual agenda is to protect the market share of the industry they are representing.

It can be difficult to tell the difference between a legitimate foundation and one dedicated only to its corporate funding. In chapter 8, I have listed some organizations that are truly independent and sincerely committed to improving your health and well-being, such as the Weston A. Price Foundation, the Institute of Science in Society, and the Union of Concerned Scientists.

It's important to adhere to the old adage "buyer beware." If you invest some time to find out the source of an organization's funding, you'll have a major clue as to their real agenda. The following is a list of several front groups for the food industry:

- **CropLife America**—originally known as the National Agricultural Chemicals Association.[42]

- **Calorie Control Council**—represents the low-calorie food industry;[43] a front group for over sixty manufacturers and suppliers that include McNeil Nutritionals (Splenda), The NutraSweet Company, Proctor & Gamble (Olestra), Tate & Lyle, Sweet'N Low, Hershey's, The Coca-Cola Company, Abbot Laboratories (Cyclamate), Pepsico Inc., and more.

- **Food Security.net**—When Graydon Forrer registered this Web site in 1999, he was the director of executive communications at Monsanto.[44] He is also an outspoken critic of organic food and farming.[45]

- **Center for Global Food Issues**—a project of the Hudson Institute, which is a think tank funded in part by agribusiness giants such as Archer Daniels Midland, ConAgra Foods, Monsanto, and Novartis.[46] The Center for Global Food Issues created a misleading "Earth Friendly, Farm Friendly" label to put on their clients' products.[47] (This is an example of labels that "use ambiguous wording to imply sustainable food production."[48])

- **Food Safety Network**—funded by the world's biggest agrochemical companies, including Dupont Canada, Eli Lilly Canada Inc., Monsanto, and Syngenta.[49]

- **International Food Information Council**—funded by Monsanto, DuPont, Frito-Lay, Coca-Cola, and NutraSweet.

- **Center for Consumer Freedom** (CCF)—a front group for the restaurant, alcohol, and tobacco industries.[50] It runs media campaigns that oppose the efforts of scientists, doctors, health advocates, and environmentalists. Anyone who criticizes tobacco, alcohol, trans fats, or soda pop is likely to come under attack from the Center for Consumer Freedom.[51] In a press release, they criticized the FDA for recommending that "U.S. restaurants reduce portion sizes, serve high calorie foods with lighter sides, advertise healthier foods and provide greater access to nutritional information."[52]

  The Center for Consumer Freedom issues press releases scoffing at the idea that mercury in fish is a problem, or that junk food contributes to obesity. Frequently, press releases such as these get aired as news with no mention of valid sources.[53, 54]

Pseudo News Designed to Deceive You

In the 1920s, Ivy Lee invented the news release.[55] Today, news releases are the vehicles by which many groups disseminate what they believe to be important information. News releases would be useful instruments if they were used to deliver truthful, constructive information, but quite often they are used to disseminate a promotional corporate agenda—in other words, they can be based more on fiction than fact. According to John Stauber, "Sometimes as many as half the stories appearing in an issue of the *Wall St. Journal* are based solely on such PR press releases."[56]

On April 6, 2006, the Center for Media and Democracy released their report "Fake TV News Widespread and Undisclosed," which exposed an epidemic of false news posing as genuine news infiltrating local television broadcasts across the country.[57] The report, written by Diane Farsetta and Daniel Price, revealed the results of a ten-month investigation of corporate-produced "video news releases," or VNRs, which have been infiltrating mainstream newscasts.[58]

Diane Farsetta, coauthor of the report, said, "It's shocking to see how product placement moves secretly unfiltered from the boardroom to the newsroom and then straight into our living rooms. Local TV broadcasts—the most popular news source in the United States—frequently air VNRs without fact-checking, conducting their own reporting, or disclosing that the footage has been provided and sponsored by big corporations."[59]

Investigators caught seventy-seven television stations actively disguising corporate-sponsored content to make it look like real news. The content came from companies including General Motors, Intel, Pfizer, and Capital One. More than one-third of the time, stations aired these self-serving, cleverly disguised public relations stories in their entirety as their own reporting.[60]

Cities with Stations Caught Airing Fake Content[61]

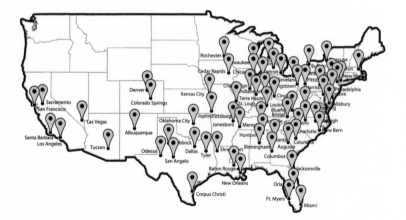

For a list of stations using fake news go to:
http://www.prwatch.org/fakenews/stationlist

Further Attempts to Eliminate
Fairness in the Media

PR firms have been pressuring networks for years; there's nothing new about that. But in the UK, PR firms have come up with a new strategy to trick unsuspecting viewers—they have been busy developing their own channels. It probably won't be long before this happens in the United States as well.

PR channels will become "infomediaries."[62] They must be able to pass themselves off as delivering real independent news, but they will offer anything but real news.

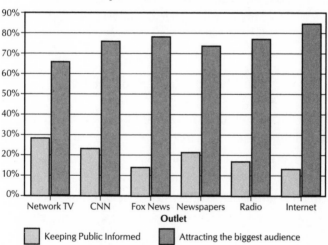

Public Perception of News Media Motives[63]

Chart created by and used with permission from Project for Excellence in Journalism, The State of the News Media, 2006. htt://www.stateofthemedia.com/2006/narrative_net-worker_publicatitudes.asp?cat=7& Media=5 based upon "Public More Critical of Press, but Goodwill Persists" from the Pew Research Center for People and the Press.

TV is not the only medium that the large corporations want to control. Currently, there is a battle going on over Internet freedom. Congress is pushing a bill that would abandon "net neutrality," the principle that preserves the free and open Internet. If it becomes law, your Internet service provider will be able to give more efficient service to sites that can afford to pay extra. Sounds fairly innocuous, doesn't it?

Except that currently, all sites on the Internet compete on a level playing field. If this we lose "net neutrality," our access to information could be severely limited. It will represent the first real battle in the coming war over Internet democracy. If the law passes, Web site owners will need to pay more for increased speed and reliability. This would enable the big players—the entrenched corporate monopolies—to overshadow the little players that frequently serve as unfiltered sources of the truth. If this law is enacted, it could easily result in a scenario that is little different than what we are witnessing today among the television networks.

You Must Learn to Spot the Lies

If we were being told the truth, we wouldn't be eating industrially processed foods (such as margarine, soy, boxed and canned foods, soda, pasteurized milk, juice, and sugar). We wouldn't have fluoride added to our water, genetically engineered crops wouldn't be growing on our planet, farmers would be farming organically, the topsoil would be rich with microbes and minerals, animals wouldn't be jailed in inhumane confinement operations, the medical system would be much more effective, and multinational drug corporations would not be one of the more lucrative industries in the world. People wouldn't need pharmaceutical drugs, as they'd be healthy from eating nutrient-dense whole foods.

With so many forms of communication, we have increased our exposure to lies and deceit. The Internet, on the one hand, has helped increase the potential to deliver honest, independent news and information. On the other hand, it has increased the possibility to spread more lies and propaganda. It is up to the viewer to be as discriminating as possible.

3

BIRD JAILS

Corporate Agribusiness and the Real Source of Bird-Borne Illness

"Food is flavored by what we know about it."
—MICHAEL POLLAN,
author of *The Omnivore's Dilemma*[1]

You've just read about how the media and their sponsors profit from a terrified audience desperate to tune in for more news. We've touched on the fact that the vaccine makers and their allies in the government are handsomely profiting, and we'll examine that in more detail in the chapter 5. But there are others that stand to benefit as well from the panic; large-scale corporate poultry operations are using the bird flu to divert attention away from their own offensive business practices and to drive their smaller rivals out of business.

It sounds unlikely, doesn't it? How could a potential panic over chicken benefit the chicken business? It sounds as strange as the panic over mad cow disease benefiting the livestock industry. Which is, of course, exactly what's happening. To get an idea of how this kind of thing works, let's take a look at the proposed National Animal Identification System (NAIS).

The National Animal Identification System

In 2002, a private membership group called the National Institute for Animal Agriculture (NIAA) cited the September 11 attacks and Bovine Spongiform Encephalopathy (BSE, or mad cow disease) as reasons to develop a nationwide, all-livestock registration tracking system.[2]

The NIAA membership includes the major U.S. meat producers (such as the National Pork Producers, Monsanto, and Cargill Meat), and the manufacturers and marketers of high-tech animal identification equipment and tracking systems (such as Digital Angel Inc., EZ-ID/AVID ID Systems, and Micro Beef Technologies Ltd.)[3]

The NIAA established private task forces to develop the plan and invited the government to take part. At some point, the USDA formally took over and continued the process.[4]

In 2005, the USDA published its plans for an animal identification system throughout the United States, a plan that is now called the National Animal Identification System. NAIS, as it is called, is a system that would require farmers to report all of their animals to a database (including horses, cows, goats, sheep, poultry, swine, llamas, alpacas, bison, elk, and deer). The government claims that the NAIS would allow it to track and control diseases in animals—such as mad cow or avian flu—more efficiently.

Sound like a good idea? Perhaps it would be . . . except that the farmers themselves are likely to be asked to take on all the costs of tracking and reporting their animals, which could include tagging their entire herd or flock with microchips or radio tags, reporting all animal movement, and buying and installing the survey system.

This isn't a problem for enormous corporate operations dealing in high-profit, low-quality, factory-farmed animals. They can afford the relatively small expense of tagging all of their livestock. Additionally, it is much easier to keep track of an animal's movement if it never leaves a crowded feedlot or spends its life crammed in a cage. But for smaller, free-range farmers, the costs will be prohibitive. With agricultural costs already at an all-time high, many small farmers will be unable to compete in this rigged marketplace and will simply be forced out of business by the onerous and costly new administrative requirements.

The USDA proposal requires that 100 percent of premises be registered by January 2009, and that all animals born after January 2008 be individually identified in order to comply with this new standard.

The USDA and agri-corporations support the claim that the NAIS is an effective strategy to "secure" your food supply.[5] They argue that, if consumers are concerned about where their meat is coming from, then this regulation would help identify the source. Superficially, this appears to make sense, but the current legislation has no provision for excluding farmers who sell directly to the consumer, or those who raise food for their own consumption. Since the source is known in these cases, they obviously do not need the "protection" of this expensive regulation. Why aren't these exceptions in the bill, if it really has to do with consumer protection, rather than eliminating small, local farmers?

Disturbing Trend In Agriculture

The United States now has more prisoners than farmers, according to the Justice Policy Institute.[6] In their 2000 report, they pointed out that there were 1,911,859 farmers in the United States, compared to 2,000,000 prisoners.

WHERE HAVE ALL OUR FARMERS GONE?[7]				
YEAR	**TOTAL POPULATION**	**FARM POPULATION**	**% OF WORK FORCE**	**AVERAGE ACRES**
1860	31,443,321	15,141,000	58%	199
1870	38,558,371	18,373,000	53%	153
1880	50,155,783	22,981,000	49%	134
1890	62,941,714	29,414,000	43%	136
1900	75,994,266	29,414,000	38%	147
1910	91,972,266	32,077,000	31%	138
1920	105,710,620	31,614,269	27%	148
1930	122,775,046	30,455,350	21%	157
1940	131,820,000	30,840,000	18%	175
1950	151,132,000	25,058,000	12.2%	216
1960	180,007,000	15,635,000	8.3%	303
1970	204,335,000	9,712,000	4.6%	390
1980	227,020,000	6,051,000	3.4%	426
1990	246,081,000	4,591,000	2.6%	461

According to the U.S. Department of Agriculture, the average net cash farm business income for farm operator households in 2004 was only $15,603.[8] That situation won't change unless consumers take initiatives, such as changing where they shop. It may take decades to rebuild local agriculture, but it won't happen unless consumers demand it. If you're concerned about food quality and keeping your family healthy, spending money at the source of the food supply—local farmers—will encourage the growth of agriculture throughout North America.

The figures in the above chart make it clear that we cannot rely on the government to encourage the growth of local farming. In fact, government policy even financially rewards landowners to NOT farm. Since 2000, the U.S. government has paid at least $1.3 billion in subsidies for rice and other crops to landowners who do no farming at all.[9] It's no mystery why we have lost so many local producers.

The U.S. Dept of Agriculture Systematically Is Destroying Independent Small Farmers

Lynn Miller, the author and publisher of *Small Farmer's Journal*, contends that the USDA "has worked for over 65 years to destroy the independent small farm community of this country. They have worked through terrible misdirected policy, deceptive loans and so-called protections/guarantees, insidious propaganda, and horrible complicity with renegade banks and unscrupulous competing agribusiness corporations."[10]

Miller believes that the NAIS could be the "most destructive and misguided farm regulation in the entire history of farming . . . This plan is patently un-American. It strikes at the very core of the Bill of Rights, the Constitution and deep into the heart of the agrarian philosophies which built this great country . . . farmers are threatened by a deep specific totalitarianism which would be comic if it weren't so ugly in consequence."[11]

Companies such as Cargill Pork and Tyson have been intimately involved in developing the NAIS program.[12] According to Judith McGeary, executive director of Farm and Ranch Freedom Alliance, Tyson has three separate individuals on the cattle working group involved in developing NAIS. "The large corporations have been the one developing the NAIS program," she adds. "The government has repeatedly told people that the working groups are supposed to represent 'the stakeholder's' interests. Yet the people making up the working groups are drawn overwhelmingly from large meat companies, technology companies, and large associations, all of whom stand to profit from NAIS."[13] McGeary and others founded the Farm and Ranch Freedom Alliance to provide a voice for the thousands of people in independent agriculture who have been ignored by the government, both in developing the NAIS and in so many other programs designed by and for industry.

Perhaps as a result of the businesses represented in the working groups, the same requirements would be imposed on a small farmer who owns 10 chickens as a large system that has 10,000 chickens, despite the differences between pastured poultry and the giant commercial operations. In fact, under the guidelines of the NAIS, large operations could apply one "tag" (or ID number) to thousands of chickens in a batch. The draft plan stipulates that in order to do this, the animals would have to be managed together from birth to death, and not comingled with other animals.

This would be practically impossible for a small farmer. Small farmers buy animals at different times of the year, and on a pastured farm, animals tend to co-mingle.

Judith McGeary describes the potential results of this scenario: Say a small farmer, who has individually identified each of his 100 pastured chickens, "finds a pile of feathers in the pasture, where a coyote or other predator carried one of the hens away. The farmer will now have to catch each of the 99 remaining chickens and note their identification numbers so that he can report which chicken has gone missing. The farmer will be faced with the option of breaking the law or spending all of his or her time simply counting the chickens."[14]

Clearly, large corporations stand to benefit by getting rid of small local farms that threaten their monopolies. Various technology companies will also profit from the NAIS. Just who will keep track of all of the animals? How will they implement the program? Who will pay for it? The NAIS will consist of many databases that will collect information from microchips or radiotags. Companies like Global Vet Link, Micro Beef Technologies, and Digital Angel are all members of the NIAA and are involved in the working groups developing the details of the plans. Such companies not only make the microchips and radiotags but charge for the software and related equipment necessary for it to function.

Is the NAIS Really Necessary?

Some might wonder whether the NAIS, despite its problems, is nonetheless necessary for disease control. Would the NAIS help control the spread of mad cow or the avian flu?

The organization Food and Water Watch doesn't think so. In an e-mail alert sent out on May 19, 2006, about the NAIS, they stated:

> Rather than devote time and resources to implementing a flawed animal identification system, Congress and USDA should be working to prevent animal diseases like mad cow disease and avian influenza that are the result of factory farm production methods. If they are sincere about gathering information necessary to track animal diseases, they should immediately fund and implement Country of Origin Labeling (C.O.O.L) for meat, which would not only give consumers information about their food, but also allow imported animals to be easily identified.[15]

Lynn Miller adds, "We have reams of scientific data that tell us without exception that by far the highest incidence of any transmittable contagion happens in industrial farm applications. That's where animals are in cramped, unhealthy conditions, and vulnerable to widespread disease outbreak."[16] If the USDA were truly interested in controlling disease they should positively reinforce the practice of raising animals in environmentally friendly surroundings and impose deterrents for inhumane animal husbandry.

Mary Zanoni, PhD, JD, and executive director of Farm for Life, sums up the views of many independent farmers: "Real food security comes from raising food yourself or buying from a local farmer you actually know. The USDA plan will only stifle local sources of production through over-regulation and unmanageable costs."[17]

It has been argued that the NAIS could help track diseases that may enter our food supply through terrorist acts.[18] But in analyzing the issue, the U.S. Government Accountability Office found that our vulnerability to animal disease, whether natural or from terrorism, stems from flaws in our food supply system that have nothing to do with identification and tracking.[19] Moreover, a system of large, consolidated farms dependent on massive shipping and transportation is far more vulnerable than a decentralized system of local farms.[20] Doug Flack, an ecologist and farmer who emphatically opposes the NAIS, says that the "NAIS will ensure that what really survives is a centralized food system, not a local food system. The safest food supply is a local food supply."[21]

Big Poultry Means Big Problems For You

Just as fears of mad cow and terrorism spawned the NAIS, large agri-corporations are using the panic over bird flu to drive yet more attempts to put small farmers out of business. But before we examine that in more detail, it might be useful to take a look at the practices of those large corporations themselves.

A market monopoly would obviously increases their bottom lines, but they have more reasons than that for seeking to instill fear about bird flu into the culture. Creating terror over unusual foreign threats, like bird flu and mad cow, helps create a distraction from their own disease-spreading practices. As the ecologists and scientists quoted above point out, it's the unhygienic practices of the large multinational corporations that are the real source of the problem here.

As the ecologists and scientists quoted above point out, it's the unhygienic practices of the large multinational corporations that are the real source of the problem.

New Methods of Raising Food

Current food production and delivery systems are dominated by only a few corporate agribusinesses, which control most of the commodity markets in corn, soybeans, and wheat, and industrial scale beef, pork, and poultry production. Their factory farming methods have been seriously compromising the human diet for the past seventy-five years.

The vast majority of traditional family farms have been replaced by the industrial farm model, which includes Concentrated Animal Feeding Operations (CAFOs). CAFOs are agricultural facilities that house and feed more than 1,000 animals in a confined area for forty-five days or more during any twelve-month period.[22] These buildings can contain many animals including cows, pigs, chickens, or turkeys.

According to a recent WorldWatch report, "State of the World 2006," "Factory farming is now the fastest growing means of animal production in the world. Industrial systems today generate:

- 74 percent of the world's poultry products,

- 50 percent of all pork,

- 43 percent of beef, and

- 68 percent of eggs."[23]

The first farm animals to be permanently confined indoors in an automated facility were chickens. According to *Broiler Industry* magazine, "Poultry became the first agribusiness because all of the factors making mechanization possible were potentially present, not the least of which was the nature of the animal itself. Relatively large number of units could be handled by a single individual, in confined areas."[24] This system also could not have been established without the use of intensive genetic selection, dietary manipulation, antibiotics, and drugs.[25]

CAFOs are a relatively new agricultural phenomenon. Fifty years ago, a typical farm might have had fewer than 100 birds; now the average chicken is raised inside a large industrial barn in groups of 5,000 to 50,000 birds.[26] In 1965, a system was developed that allowed one person to operate a plant producing 40,000 birds a day.[27]

A broiler chicken is raised for its meat; a hen is a layer chicken used for producing eggs. In order to increase production and reduce costs, laying hens or broiler chickens are clustered together like sardines in these bird jails and are force-fed foods they would most likely never eat in the wild. CAFOs represent a radical departure from the days when animals were left outside on green pastures basking in the sun and grazing on lush grass.

In 2004, the U.S. produced 8.7 billion broiler chickens—about a 65 percent increase over the previous fourteen years.[28] On average, Americans now eat 250 percent more chicken than they did forty years ago. Our increase in demand for chicken, however, has come with heavy environmental, health, and economic burdens.

INCREASE IN CHICKEN CONSUMPTION	
YEAR	POUNDS/PERSON/YEAR
1966	32.1[29]
1970	40.1[30]
2000	81.2[31]

Factory Farming Increases Bird Diseases

In 2005, WorldWatch published the report "Happier Meals: Rethinking the Global Meat Industry." The author of the report, Danielle Nierenberg, points out that when birds are raised in unhygienic confinement operations, they are more susceptible to illness.[32]

In order to maximize production, confinement animals are forced to remain indoors, away from the natural light of the sun, fresh air, and the opportunity to consume the fresh plants and insects that are part of their normal diet. Depriving the animals of these essential requirements to stay healthy is an absolute prescription for disaster. Nierenberg warns, "Crowded and unhygienic conditions can sicken farm animals and create the perfect environment for the spread of diseases, including outbreaks of avian flu, bovine spongiform encephalopathy (BSE), and foot-and-mouth disease."[33]

CAFOs and Bird Flu

GRAIN's report "Fowl Play: The Poultry Industry's Central Role in the Bird Flu Crisis," points out that there is growing evidence that highly infectious bird flu actually originates in Concentrated Animal Feeding Operations, and is more than likely spread by the globalized poultry trade.[34] The media tends to paint a different picture, implicating wild birds or small backyard poultry operations as being the source of the highly pathogenic bird flu virus. However, blaming backyard poultry or migratory birds simply doesn't make sense, as small outdoor flocks of birds have a better chance of keeping viral loads down. If a highly infectious bird flu virus were to infect and kill all the birds in a small flock, the virus likely wouldn't spread and infect other birds.

On the other hand, in a CAFO with a high density of birds, the H5N1 virus can spread and multiply very quickly. Transporting the birds, eggs, and other by-products from these facilities can further increase the risk of spreading the disease.

Dr. Shiv Chopra is a microbiologist and worked as a drug evaluator at Health Canada for thirty-five years, until he was suddenly fired. Thanks to his efforts, bovine growth hormone, rBGH, was not approved for use in dairy cows in Canada. He has spoken out about the dangers of hormones, antibiotics, and feeding animal by-products to food-producing animals, and he is presently writing a book, about his experiences while working for the Canadian government.

Dr. Chopra, who is also a veterinarian, thinks the CAFOs bear responsibility for spreading bird illness: "Chickens raised in an artificial environment (factory farming) are more prone to get sick with various infections, including with bird flu. When you feed animals garbage, containing all kinds of chemicals and dead animal parts, and put them together in intense concentrations, they are bound to get sick. That is what happens."[35]

According to the World Health Organization, "Piled one on top of the other in cramped cages, [factory farmed] birds easily pass the disease on with their dirty droppings."[36] Dr. Walter Sontag, an Austrian zoologist who has studied the H5N1 virus, points out that "a high density [of birds] in a small space with defined food and water availability, and in addition, poor hygiene conditions promote an explosive spread of pathogenic germ cells."[37]

Wendy Orent, author of *Plague: The Mysterious Past and Terrifying Future of the World's Most Dangerous Disease*, writes that

> . . . lethal bird flu is entirely man-made . . . People have been living with backyard flocks of poultry since the dawn of civilization. But it wasn't until poultry production became modernized, and birds were raised in much larger numbers and concentrations, that a virulent bird flu evolved. When birds are packed close together, any brakes on virulence are off.[38]

Humans who are in close contact with these sick chickens can also contract the bird flu virus. In Turkey, three children died from the

H5N1 virus after they were exposed to sick and dying birds that came from a local CAFO.[39]

Southeastern and central Asian countries have expanded their poultry industry dramatically over the last ten years or so. In Thailand, Indonesia, and Vietnam, production of chicken meat jumped from approximately 300,000 metric tonnes in 1971 to 2,440,000 tonnes in 2001.[40] In China, chicken production tripled during the 1990s', to over 9 million tonnes a year.[41] Most of the new poultry production in these countries has been centered around CAFOs, which are built outside of major cities and are part of the transnational production system.

As you can see by the charts below, the rapid growth in the China's poultry industry seems to correspond with the increase in the numbers of cases of the H5N1 virus. The highly pathogenic avian influenza virus H5N1 first caused disease in Hong Kong in 1997, infecting eighteen patients and causing six deaths. The virus, then, seemed to surface along with the increase in China poultry production.

Increase in Asian Chicken Production[42]
Ready-to-Cook Thousands of Metric Tons

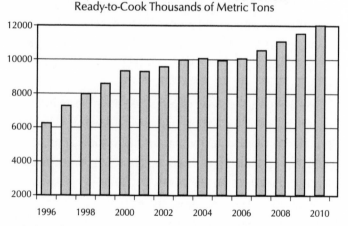

Dr. Paul Aho, The Outlook for Asian Feed Demand, USDA Agricultural Outlook Forum, February 17, 2006
http://www.usda.gov/oce/forum/2006%20Speeches/PDF%20PPT/Aho.pdf

Increase in Asian Chicken Production[43]

CHICKEN PRODUCTION IN MMT*, 1984–2004			
	1984	2004	2024
Asia	6	21	42
United States	6	16	24
World	26	68	120
Asia % of World Supply	23%	31%	35%

*(Millions of Metric Tons)

Dr. Paul Aho, The Outlook for Asian Feed Demand, USDA Agricultural Outlook Forum, February 17, 2006
http://www.usda.gov/oce/forum/2006%20Speeches/PDF%20PPT/Aho.pdf

The UN's Food and Agriculture Organization (FAO) has stated that "the major factors contributing to the spread of the bird flu virus are poor hygienic practices related to the production, processing and marketing of poultry, contaminated products, gaps in biosecurity and individuals not following recommended control measures."[44] But even though the FAO has made this statement, they have not done an adequate job of monitoring or regulating the unhygienic practices of factory farming, including the practice of feeding chicken manure to fish farms.

Billions of Pounds of poultry Manure May Be the REAL Source of Bird Flu

The practice of using chicken manure as fish feed or fertilizer on certain crops is creating the same threat as feeding animal by-products to cattle. This time the threat is the H5N1 highly pathogenic bird flu.

The chicken industry makes a great deal of money off the sale of by-products (such as manure, blood, bones, liver, lung) rendered from processing birds. Chicken manure from factory farms is a potentially infectious and toxic nightmare. It can contain campy-lobacter, salmonella, parasites, veterinary drug residues, and toxic heavy metals such as arsenic, lead, cadmium and mercury, as well as the bird flu virus itself.[45, 46]

Since chicken manure (even millions of pounds of chicken manure sitting dormant in a lagoon) is not classified as a "hazardous waste," it can be sold and re-used for other purposes. Conveniently for the corporations, manure simply doesn't fit under any clearly defined rules, making it difficult to regulate even though it is very clearly a "hazardous" substance. Approximately 90 percent of the waste is currently applied to fields and cropland as fertilizer.[47] It can also be fed to cattle and, as mentioned above, fish in fish farms. In January 2004, the FDA proposed banning the practice; however, in October 2005, they changed their minds and allowed it to continue.[48]

Even though they sell the manure, the factory chicken farms are producing more waste than they can get rid of. In the United States, these bird jails generate between 26 and 55 billion pounds of waste annually, which has created an enormous environmental burden in certain areas. In Arkansas alone, chicken farms produce an amount of waste each day equal to that produced by 8 million people.[49]

> **Manure simply doesn't fit under any defined rules, making it difficult to regulate even though it is clearly very hazardous.**

One of the largest sources of polluted runoff comes from factory farms.[50] Homeowners who live downwind from CAFO facilities not only have to put up with their horrible stench, they also have to tolerate reduced property value. How would you like to live downwind from a factory farm? In 2005, Oklahoma attorney general Drew Edmondson filed suit against Tyson, Cargill, and several other poultry companies, seeking to stop water pollution caused in his state by chicken waste dumped in Arkansas.[51]

In Prairie Grove, Arkansas, a small town where cancer rates are fifty times higher than the national average, a group of citizens filed a lawsuit against several poultry producers for damages from arsenic-contaminated chicken manure spread as fertilizer.[52] The poultry companies being sued are Alpharma, Alpharma Animal Health, Cal-Maine Farms, Cargill, George's Peterson, Simmons, and Tyson Foods. As of June 21, 2006, the lawsuit is still ongoing, and the poultry companies are trying to get the case dismissed.[53]

When Fish Are Fed Chicken Manure, Bad Things Happen

Poultry manure is commonly used in commercial freshwater aquaculture, as it acts as a fertilizer and helps to stimulate the growth of the fish. In nature, fish don't eat rendered chicken parts or chicken manure, nor do they ear canola or soy (another common practice in the commercial fish industry). This practice presents a potential risk for the spread of any disease, including the highly pathogenic bird flu. Since the H5N1 virus can live for several days in moisture, it is possible that the virus could be spread by chicken manure or even chicken by-products.

Professor Chris Feare, author of the report "Fish Farming and the Risk of Spread of Avian Influenza," points a few instances where birds have been found dead near fish farms. For example, in October 2005, "the deaths of Mute Swans *Cygnus olor* in the two [avian flu] outbreaks in Croatia both occurred at fish farms."[54] At Lake Qinghai in China, thousands of wild birds died from the highly infectious bird flu—they were found near fish farms that allegedly use feed containing chicken manure.

> **"The deaths of Mute Swans . . . in the two [avian flu] outbreaks in Croatia both occurred at fish farms."**
> —PROFESSOR CHRIS FEARE

In an FAO report from 2003 on "Integrated Livestock-Fish Farming Systems," they noted that "recently, livestock and fish have been implicated in the irregular occurrence of influenza pandemics; the global impacts on public health of promoting livestock and fish integration are huge if these claims are substantiated."[55] On December 28, 2005, however, FAO chief veterinary officer Joseph Domenech contradicted the 2003 report, dismissing the idea that the widespread use of poultry excrement to fertilize fish farms posed a serious danger.[56] But scientific studies have recognized the practice as a risk for spreading avian flu pandemics.[57]

Conservationist Dr. Martin Williams has traveled to Indonesia and reported on the appalling conditions of some of the "integrated fish farming" operations:[58]

> I have been involved in discussions regarding the possibility "integrated fish farming" may play a role in sustaining and even spreading H5N1 bird flu: including when poultry manure is used as fish feed . . . So when I stayed by a fish farm just outside Jakarta at the beginning of this month, I took a walk around.
>
> Surprised by what I saw—included chicken carcasses being devoured by catfish. Carcasses, and bags of poultry manure, perhaps from an adjoining chicken farm, which was in a walled compound with a guard post at the gate. Took several photos, several of which are below: warning, not too great if you're squeamish, or perhaps about to eat.[58]

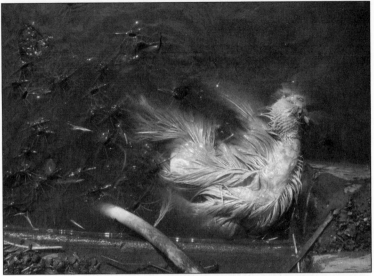

The fish were feeding very actively, on dead chickens floating by edge of the pond. Now, suppose chickens had died of H5N1. Surely this way, would get H5N1 into the fish guts (how long might it remain?), as well as onto skin, and into water. (Images used courtesy of www.drmartinwilliams.com)

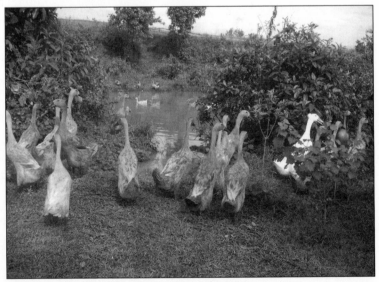

Just beside the fishponds was this small duck pond.

The use of fresh manure from farm animals as feed for fish ponds is a common practice in Asia and central Europe.[59] And, because many migratory birds have been found dead near fish farming operations in those areas, Bird Life International is now calling for an investigation into the possibility that these thousands of manure-fed ponds may be the means by which the H5N1 bird flu virus is being spread. There have been several reports of migratory birds found dead near fish farming operations.[60] Further investigation is required to find out if these farms were feeding chicken manure to the fish, whether the manure is treated for potential contaminants, and where the manure came from.

They Are Feeding Arsenic to Your Chickens!

Arsenic has been touted as being the "king of poisons".[61] Long-term exposure to arsenic puts you at risk of developing cancer of the skin, bladder, kidney, liver, lung, colon, uterus, prostate, and stomach, as well as diabetes mellitus and vascular, reproductive, developmental and neurological effects.[62] Arsenic has also been shown to be a powerful endocrine disruptor.[63]

David Wallinga is the director of the Institute for Agriculture and Trade Policy's (IATP) food and health program. He is the author of the report "Playing Chicken: Avoiding Arsenic in Your Meat." Minneapolis-based IATP tested 155 samples from uncooked supermarket chicken products. They found that 55 percent carried detectable arsenic.[64]

Arsenic is used as a growth promoter in industrial poultry production systems. Some of it is retained in the meat and converted to more toxic forms, adding to your total arsenic intake. Arsenic in chicken manure may also migrate to groundwater, and if the manure is used as fertilizer, possibly to food crops. Arsenic levels in

U.S. long-grain rice were the highest found in a recent survey of rice from different countries.[65]

The use of arsenic as a feed supplement is banned in Europe, but the U.S. FDA has failed to ban this toxic substance. Of the 8.7 billion American broiler chickens produced each year, estimates are that at least 70 percent have been fed arsenic.[66]

The results of tests conducted on chicken breasts by the IATP showed that the highest level measured was at 21.2 parts per billion.[67] The poultry industry claims that the arsenic levels found in chicken are so low consumers have nothing to worry about. But the EPA has determined that the safety standard of arsenic in water is 10 parts per billion.[68]

Movie Reveals Shocking Practices

Animal rights activists have been working to expose other atrocities associated with the practice of factory farming. A large U.S. grocery chain, Wegmans, built their first egg farm in 1967, which was considered the world's largest at that time. Their current egg farm has the capacity for seven hundred thousand birds. A recent undercover operation by an organization called Compassionate Consumers investigated the abominable conditions under which chickens were being raised at the egg farm. The results of their investigation can be seen online in their video *Wegmans Cruelty* at www.greatbirdfluhoax.com/wegmans.[69]

They found up to nine hens living in a space the size of a filing cabinet. In conventional egg production, hens live in what are called "battery" cages, which means that several are stacked on top of each other. The hens are already so crowded that they sometimes have to stand on each other. And with cages piled on top of each other, the excrement of the hens from above lands on those below. Investigators describe the smell in the Wegmans facility as being "unbearable".[70]

However, somehow these conditions do not preclude Wegmans from using an "Animal Care Certified" logo on each package of eggs that they sell. This logo is considered misleading by organizations including the Better Business Bureau, which says that the egg industry should stop advertising their product as being "humane."[71,72] Miyun Park, a former investigator with Compassion Over Killing, explains, "The cruelty is inherent in battery cage production. There is no way to raise and care for a hen humanely in these conditions."[73]

> "The egg industry should stop advertising its products as humane as long as it continues such practices as clipping hens' beaks and depriving birds of food and water . . ."
> —The Better Business Bureau (2004)[74, 75]

In early May 2006, the maker of the film *Wegmans Cruelty*, Adam Durand, was sentenced for trespassing on Wegmans egg farm in Wayne County, New York. His convictions earned him 180 days in jail, $1,500 in fines, a year of probation, and 100 hours of community service.[76] It is no surprise that the lobby group Center for Consumer Freedom (CCF), which is a front group for the restaurant, alcohol, and tobacco industries,[77] supported the sentence, calling Durand a "low level criminal".[78]

To date, however, charges were never brought against Wegmans, even though the film provides evidence that they may have violated the law. The film shows that some of the laying hens did not have access to water because their necks were stuck in the cage, preventing them from reaching their water source. It is shocking that this type of abuse of animal conditions and deceitful advertising can persist without penalty.

For years now, many animal activist groups have been trying

to expose and stop the inhumane practices going on in these "bird jails." Animal activists have good intentions, but the real solution to this problem is to change supply and demand by educating consumers to change where they shop. In turn, this will help reduce the chance of spreading diseases such as the highly pathogenic bird flu.

Factory Farm Workers
Develop Health Problems

Workers who are subjected to the filthy conditions within these factory farms have reported a variety of health problems. Workers who spend long hours in factory farms can develop asthma and allergic pneumonitis.[79] In large enclosed dairy farming operations, there is also an increased incidence of "farmer's lung" disease.[80]

Ellen Silbergeld, professor of environmental science at the Johns Hopkins Bloomberg School of Public Health, has stated that "people who are in contact with live poultry have increased health issues and they are more likely to be carrying drug-resistant bacteria compared to [other] people in the community."[81] Keep in mind that a number of those who have contracted the highly pathogenic H5N1 virus have been in close contact with sick poultry from factory farms.

Furthermore, Dr. Silbergeld's research indicates that:

- "Chicken catchers had significantly more symptoms of neurological problems, such as paralysis and muscle weakness, compared with others."

- ". . . poultry workers exhibited more symptoms of gastrointestinal illnesses, such as diarrhea, because of exposure to campylobacter, a bacteria found often in poultry."[82]

The employees who work inside these operations are suffering the health consequences from being exposed to dander, dust, micro-organisms (disease), arsenic, ammonia, and other chemicals found in feed and manure. According to Jennifer Rosenbaum, a lawyer with the Southern Poverty Law Center, "There are huge health and safety violations in every plant."[83] In 2004, the Occupational Safety and Health Administration (OSHA) issued citations to Tyson for alleged violations after an employee was asphyxiated when he inhaled hydrogen sulfide, a gas created by decaying organic matter.[84]

Vertical Integration

The real disease the world is facing is not bird flu, but something called vertical integration, a system which consists of a few corporations controlling the entire food chain. Within this system, a single company can sell seed to the farmer, operate the local grain elevator, own the railroad and the port facility, buy the grain from the farmer, and sell the grain to itself to be processed into food.[85]

Through vertical integration, corporations like Tyson are able to take control of every stage of the chicken production process:

- Genetics
- Chicken hatching
- Feed manufacturing
- Chicken processing
- Advertising
- Exporting transportation
- Value-added chicken products[86]

Vertical integration has been a boon for a few very powerful players in the food industry, but it has driven many small farmers out of business because they simply can't compete with the control of the large corporations. And that allows those corporations to get away with any practices, however harmful, that they think might increase their bottom lines; the lack of alternatives keeps consumers from going elsewhere.

Vertical integration allows a few companies to maximize their profits, while ignoring both the health of the animals and the health of the people who purchase their food. According to Charles Margulis, a spokesperson for the Center for Food Safety, "As the experience with mad cow disease shows, most factory farming corporations tend to ignore food quality issues until there is some adverse effect related to their bottom line."[87]

The highly pathogenic strain of bird flu has emerged along with the growth of industrialized poultry farming. While the bird flu will never be a pandemic, it has killed over one hundred people and is threatening the lives of millions of birds. The unhygienic conditions in the factory farms threaten the quality and safety of all products that emerge from this environment. Such is the case with poultry by-products (manure, bones, blood, guts, feathers, and dead birds, for example) that are sold from these mammoth operations.

An article published in one of the most prestigious scientific journals, *Science*, states that "for the H5N1 virus, it is without doubt that domestic waterfowl, specific farming practices, and agro-ecological environments played a key role in the occurrence, maintenance, and spread of HPAI for many affected countries . . ."[88]

As long as there is evidence suggesting that factory farming is somehow involved in the spread of the highly pathogenic bird flu, by making birds sick and then selling the birds, meat, eggs, or by-products such as manure, officials should be at a minimum demanding further investigation into the matter. Currently, however, I do not believe officials are doing enough to address the problem.

As long as officials don't draw attention to factory farming as a potential source of the highly pathogenic bird flu virus, mainstream media will also ignore the issue. Some stories in the media have even pointed to the smuggled bird trade, fighting cocks and tropical pets as being potential causes for the spread of the deadly bird flu. They seem to use every means imaginable to distract people from learning that factory farming has anything to do with the highly pathogenic bird flu. Instead, the blame is being laid elsewhere.

4

SHIFTING THE BLAME

How the Big Poultry Companies Make Money from the Bird Flu Scare

Enormous efforts have taken place in order to prove that migratory birds are the cause of the spread of the highly infectious avian flu. Practically every news story on the subject has talked of the risk of migrating birds carrying the disease from country to country. In May 2006, as part of an attempt to prove the theory that migratory birds are to blame, 15,000 birds were tested in Alaska, at a cost of about $4 million.[1] Thousands of wild birds have also been tested in other parts of the world.

But even after such great effort and expense, little evidence has been found to support the theory. According to veterinarian Richard Slemons, a bird-flu expert at Ohio State University, the evidence that wild birds are involved in spreading the virus is circumstantial at best.[2] Birdlife International's Dr. Richard Thomas says, "when plotted, the pattern of outbreaks follows major road and rail routes, not flyways."[3]

In a press release dated July 16, 2004, the UN's Food and Agriculture Organization urged countries in Asia not to destroy wild birds. According to Juan Lubroth of the FAO Animal Health Service, "Killing wild birds will not help to prevent or control avian influenza outbreaks . . . to date, there is no scientific evidence that wildlife is the major factor in the resurgence of the disease in the region."[4]

> According to Juan Lubroth of the FAO Animal Health Service, "Killing wild birds will not help to prevent or control avian influenza outbreaks . . . to date, there is no scientific evidence that wildlife is the major factor in the resurgence of the disease in the region."

The Royal Society for the Protection of Birds told the BBC that the trade in birds and the movement of poultry products is more likely the cause of the spread of H5N1.[5] Almost all of the wild birds that have tested positive for the disease were already dead and, in most cases, found near outbreaks in domestic poultry.[6]

Wild birds and poultry in Asia, Turkey and Nigeria that have fallen victim to the highly infectious bird flu appear to have been exposed to birds from CAFOs. For example, Nigeria, where the first outbreak of highly infectious bird flu occurred in Africa, imports live birds and feed (which contains chicken manure) from CAFOs located in China.

But the CAFOs seldom get mentioned in news stories. The media's favorite target appears to be migratory birds, however. Sometimes they happen to mention that outbreaks have been linked to other sources, such as the illegal trade in poultry and/or caged birds, or live animal markets, where domestic and wild-caught birds are kept in close proximity.[7]

Factory Farming Goal is to Eliminate Backyard Farms

We have finally come full circle, to the method the large poultry corporations are using to make bird flu a wedge to drive their smaller competitors out of business. Rather than correcting the hygiene conditions on the big CAFOs, they are diverting attention to small farms. It is there, they argue, that bird flu lurks. They claim that birds put outdoors in their natural environment, rather than being crammed in cages for their entire lives, are at greater risk of catching bird flu from migrating birds. Major chicken producers such as Tyson, Perdue, and ConAgra are all developing disinformation campaigns stating that their chickens are "safer" because they are "inside."[8] But the irony is that outdoor poultry are actually far more likely to be healthy than poultry from indoor operations that house thousands of birds together.

In an area where nearby farms were affected by the bird flu, an organic farmer in Buriman, Veerapon Sopa, announced that his outdoor flock of about one hundred chickens, forty ducks, and a few geese weren't infected with the virus. He believes that his pastured poultry have a stronger immune system that helps protect them from disease.[9]

A farm operator in Ang Thong Thailand also doesn't support the idea that enclosing poultry in a building is healthier for the birds. He was quoted in the Bangkok Post as saying, "Ms. Chatamas had operated a closed-farm for five years and through her experience had found that the number of chickens which had died from avian flu in her closed farm was higher than those in open farms, due to lack of immunity."[10]

Exposure to sunlight produces many powerful immune boosting benefits, and prior to the advent of antibiotics was one of the few effective treatment options for the treatment of tuberculosis.[11] Evidence published earlier this year in *Science* supports the idea that sunlight-produced vitamin D triggers a powerful antimicrobial response.[12]

Now in fact, some small farms do contribute to the spread of diseases like bird flu—but not for the reason being claimed. The problem is that conditions on small farms in some parts of the world can be unhygienic. At night, to prevent theft, family farmers bring the poultry in their homes, where they may roost on the kitchen sink and faucet. In some cases, residents even sleep in close proximity to these birds.

So, just as the NAIS actually would help to track disease, while driving most small farms out of business, eliminating small poultry farms might indeed do something to help stop the spread of bird-borne illness . . . while completely eliminating any rivals to the big poultry companies.

In addition, not all outdoor farming operations are created equal. Joel Salatin, author of *Holy Cows and Hog Heaven*, calls himself an "honest-to-goodness-dirt-under-the-fingernails, optimistic clean food farmer." Before the media tries to blame all backyard poultry operators for spreading the bird flu, Salatin insists, "Perhaps they need to brush up on the differences between a clean and a filthy outdoor operation."[13]

It is not unreasonable to ask any farming operation to practice sound hygiene. In technical terms, it's called "bio-security." Farmers know that their animals can get sick, and most will take reasonable hygienic measure to make sure that their farm is "bio-secure." But the measures that have imposed on farms in an attempt to address the bird flu dilemma present an unaffordable expense to most small farmers, such as enclosing the birds in nets or buildings, or destroying the birds wholesale.

Sound familiar?

Instead of threatening the livelihoods of millions of families who own backyard poultry flocks, perhaps concerned governments should consider educating the families that operate these backyard operations about better hygiene. That would stop the spread of disease without driving the farms out of business—if that is the actual goal.

GRAIN's report "Fowl Play: The Poultry Industry's Central Role in the Bird Flu Crisis" provides several examples of H5N1 outbreaks that occurred in factory farm settings. But whenever there is an outbreak, culling programs are indiscriminate and include backyard poultry along with the chicken from industrial operations. Poultry from small backyard operations can be killed simply because they are within a certain distance of the outbreak. Essentially, poultry from small flocks have frequently become "innocent bystanders."

In 2004, over thirty-five commercial poultry operations were infected with an avian flu virus (H7N3) in British Columbia, Canada. Not only were the majority of nearby outdoor flocks healthy, they did not even carry any antibodies for the avian flu. But the Canadian Food Inspection Agency (CFIA) culled millions of birds, both from outdoor and indoor operations. The area in British Columbia that experienced the outbreak has a large number of regular broiler barns, turkey barns, and commercial layer operations built in close proximity to each other. According to Stella Purdy, president of the Fraser Valley Poultry Fanciers Association, "Any health professional can tell you that it is a disaster waiting to happen."[14]

Several small poultry producers thought that the CFIA's culling operation was needless, given that their birds tested negative for the bird flu virus. Many small poultry operations resisted the CFIA's attempts to destroy their birds. Purdy explained that the CFIA even admitted that they needed to strong arm the situation for political and economic reasons: "It was explained over and over to me that the reason the kill had to go forward even though it was obviously not going to work was because that way Canada would be perceived by the rest of the world as having a decisive policy and thereby keep its trading place in commerce."[15]

As millions of birds have been killed, factory farms have been compensated for their losses. The small farmers, whose lives depend on revenues from the regular sale of their poultry, are also promised compensation, but payments are frequently delayed, causing serious cash flow problems that threaten the solvency of these small businesses. In some cases, there have been reports that farmers may not be compensated at all.[16] The World Health Organization has noted resistance among small farmers to culling operation as a result of the "frequent absence of compensation . . . for destroyed birds."[17]

Ganesh Sonar, a farmer in Navapur, Maharashtra, India, pointed out the irony of attention being paid to small farms as a result of the bird flu scare: "We live in poverty, without any basic facilities and no one coming to enquire about our problems. All of a sudden all the television crews, media persons and doctors wearing surgical masks are roaming our dirt roads to collect more statistics. Our chickens were our only source of income and now they have destroyed even that. Is this what is called governance?"[18]

With the responsibility for the spread of the highly pathogenic bird flu being directed toward "outdoor" birds, officials are moving to "restructure" the poultry industry by imposing unrealistic restrictions on backyard flocks.[19] According to Margaret Say, Southeastern Asian director for the USA Poultry and Egg Export Council, "We cannot control migratory birds but we can surely work hard to close down as many backyard farms as possible."[20]

The adverse media exposure about these small farms has resulted in a 30–40 percent decrease in demand for live birds.[21] (In contrast, the general global drop in demand for poultry as a result of bird flu has been 3 percent.) This is not an insignificant issue; you might be surprised to learn that the Live Bird Markets, which target sales to the poorest half of the world's population, represent $20 billion in world retail sales, and involve 40 million small farms in Asia.[22] The Live Bird Markets are also important to the poor, as many of them cannot afford refrigeration. Even though the livelihoods of millions of Asians rely on the sale of Live Bird Markets, as the graph below shows it is predicted that the live bird market will decline while the commercial chicken industry increases. Bear in mind that millions of Asians do not have the money to buy a refrigerator, and so are in much greater danger of eating spoiled meat if they are forced to buy chicken from retail stores rather than slaughtering fresh chicken themselves.

Cold Chain &Live Market Consumption [23] Per Capita–Lbs.

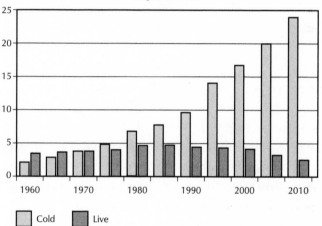

Dr. Paul Aho, The Outlook for Asian Feed Demand, USDA Agricultural Outlook Forum, February 17, 2006
http://www.usda.gov/oce/forum/2006%20Speeches/PDF%20PPT/Aho.pdf

Even with the real need for hygiene and bio-security education, blaming the backyard farms is nothing but a distraction from the real source of the problem. According to Dr. Mae-Wan Ho, when a team of scientists analyzed the H5N1 epidemic in Thailand in 2004, they found that the risks for highly infectious bird flu infection were up to 32.4 times higher for commercial birds than for backyard chickens.[24, 25]

She adds, "This is clear evidence . . . that supports other findings that industrial poultry corporate factory farms are to blame, responsible for spreading the bird flu virus, and not independent small backyard farms. On that basis, we should be calling for closure of factory farms, not family farms."[26]

> "This is clear evidence . . . that supports other findings that industrial poultry corporate factory farms are to blame, responsible for spreading the bird flu virus, and not independent small backyard farms."
>
> —DR. MAE-WAN HO

What's Good For the Goose Is Good for the Gander?

Perhaps large poultry corporations should be more critical of their own system, and perhaps government inspectors should be more critical of large poultry operations than of small backyard flocks. In 2002, Joel Salatin, one of America's premier grass farmers, witnessed an avian flu outbreak in Shenandoah Valley Virginia, where there are several "bird jails." Several million chickens and turkeys were destroyed in order to prevent the spread of the virus, which was the H7N2 variety.

Salatin recalls that during the outbreak, an official announced that "one single" feather carried enough virus to infect 500,000 birds. "Just drive down the interstate and ask yourself how we could survive after being exposed to all the feathers falling out of a tractor trailer load of chickens."[27] When he drove behind trucks carrying poultry parts (bones, beaks, claws, etc . . .), the parts fell off of the trucks and hit his windshield like shrapnel. And for miles outside of the processing plants, Salatin could see chicken feathers scattered in ditches.[28]

If a feather could be carrying a virus, then what are they doing about their own bio-security in the ditches around their plants and on the roads during the transportation of chickens or their body parts? If they are really serious about preventing the spread of any virus, then factory farms and their transportation vehicles need to be hermetically sealed.

The irony is that pastured poultry from local farms are much less of a bio-security risk than chickens that are transported for hundreds of miles in trucks. Salatin, who processes his chickens right on the farm, confirms that "our feathers stay right here."[29]

If the bird flu does influence the nature of the poultry industry, all pastured poultry producers could be adversely affected. Depending upon how bio-security measures are enforced, and whether the NAIS imposes the tracking of farm animals, many small producers could be driven out of business. The bio-security measures for pastured poultry could include a requirement that the birds be covered by a net at all times. Most small producers probably wouldn't have the money to pay for a large net to cover their flocks.

The same would not be true for the large poultry operations. This is simply not a level playing field! The pastured poultry producers could soon be fighting for their survival.

Who is Profiting from the Panic?

In 2004, the Food and Agriculture Organization (FAO) released a report indicating that the impact of the economic losses resulting from the bird flu far outweighed the rare human deaths. According to the report, "The impact of countries banning both Thai and Chinese poultry exports are leading to higher international poultry prices and increasing demand for poultry meat from other major suppliers, such as the United States . . ."[30]

In other words, large U.S. chicken producers are profiting from the economic losses in Asia. They have been anxious to tap into the Asian market, which represents 7 billion chickens, 40 percent of the global production.[31]

Since the bird flu scare, many countries have imposed bans on importing chicken from countries where outbreaks have occurred. For example, Japan (which imports approximately 70 percent of its chicken) has imposed a ban on chicken imports from Thailand and China. Many countries that have had outbreaks of the highly pathogenic bird flu have lost millions of dollars in exports.

Bans have forced some countries to import chicken from the United States and Brazil, resulting in huge profits for companies such as Tyson, Perdue, and ConAgra.[32] Tyson has a history of taking advantage of any disaster that befalls its competitors. In 1997, when Hudson Foods was hit with an E. coli scandal, Tyson was waiting in ready to buy the company at a rock bottom price. A few years later, in 2001, an outbreak of foot-and-mouth disease in the UK resulted in the destruction of approximately 7 million sheep and cattle, costing Britain £8 billion ($15 billion U.S.). As a result, IBP Inc., a large meat packing company, experienced an enormous decrease in profits. It was promptly acquired by Tyson Foods in 2001 for $3.2 billion in cash and stock. By "rescuing" IBP from their plight, Tyson increased their control of the beef, chicken, and pork markets.

Another company that stands to benefit from the panic over "outdoor" birds is the Bangkok-based poultry giant Charoen Pokphand (CP). CP is a massive Thai enterprise that owns a major chunk of poultry production throughout Thailand and China, as well as in Indonesia, Cambodia, Vietnam, and Turkey. They exported about 270 million chickens in 2003 alone.[33] The chairman of the CP Group, Dhanin Chearavanont, has been claiming that CP's closed facilities are safer than backyard ones.[34]

Interestingly, however, the Thai government admitted the presence of the virus in CP facilities on January 23, 2004. Officials in Thailand withheld this information for two months prior to the announcement.[35] During that period, workers in the industry were told to accelerate the processing of the chickens after they noticed signs of disease: "Before November we were processing about 90,000 chickens a day," a worker in a poultry factory recalled, "but from November to 23 January, we had to kill about 130,000 daily."[36]

Government Policies
Discriminate Against Small Farms

In Canada, certain government policies support the large poultry producers and impose unrealistic restrictions on small producers. On September 12, 2005, the Ottawa Citizen reported on a farmers' protest at the Perth Farmer's Market in Canada. Farmers were expecting a confrontation with government officials after they showed up at the market for the regular sale of their farm fresh eggs. If "caught" selling eggs, they risked being fined $5,000.[37] Health inspectors had dredged up an old federal law stating that "eggs must be graded at a grading station that had been approved by the Canadian Food Inspection Agency or build a federally-approved official egg grading station on their farms."[38]

Bear in mind that egg grading does not identify unsafe eggs, so cannot affect health or safety. As Maureen Bostock of Sweet Meadow Farm points out, "Egg grading . . . has nothing to do with protecting consumers from food-borne disease."[39] It was simply an excuse to keep the farmers from bringing their eggs to market.

In Perth, there's only one federally approved grading station— and it doesn't accept eggs from small local vendors.[40] And those small local farmers also can't afford to buy sophisticated systems that candle, weigh, disinfect, and coat eggs with a preservative to prolong shelf-life—all of which requires a "separate facility with two refrigerators, special sinks, solutions to rinse eggs and even a white uniform for the farmer to wear while grading the eggs."[41]

The health inspectors were happy to approve the sale of canned pop, popsicles, Mr. Freeze, potato chips, and chewing gum at the farmer's market, incidentally.

The inspectors finally did back down in this particular case. But the incident demonstrates a disturbing tendency. A European Commission poll showed that almost 50 percent of European citizens believe the authorities favor economic interests over consumer health, and they no longer believe what the regulators say.[42] In fact they are so disillusioned by what the authorities say that they tend to believe just the opposite of what the regulators tell them.[43]

This behavior cannot be allowed to continue. If the big companies, and the government organizations they lobby so extensively, are able to accelerate the dissolution of small farms, then the only poultry choice you will have will be unhealthy, factory-farmed birds.

Can You Spot the Deceptions?

Reports do point out that the majority of people who have been infected with H5N1 have been in close contact with sick poultry. However, what you're not necessarily being told is where these poultry are coming from.

Billions of dollars are spent annually on press releases that are designed to protect the interests of the groups releasing them. (On February 13, 2006, it was announced that the Bush Administration spent over $1.6 billion on advertising and public relations contracts since 2003.[44]) Many of these press releases are not designed to inform you; rather they are designed to distract you from learning the real truth.

When you hear stories about the bird flu, consider that many details have been conveniently being left out. It is in the best interest of certain groups to divert your attention away from the controversial problems behind the bird flu. The path to finding the root cause of the problem is learning to ask the right questions. The question to ask in this case is not about flu viruses in wild birds but about the conditions in which commercial birds are being raised.

Perhaps Florence Nightingale said it best: "The specific disease doctrine is the grand refuge of weak, uncultured, unstable minds, such as now rule in the medical profession. There are no specific diseases; there are specific disease conditions."[45]

In other words, disease is more strongly related to diet, lifestyle and the environment than to the "germ" that is being blamed for the disease. The mainstream media, along with the majority of the medical profession, have somehow forgotten this important doctrine and routinely ignore stories that focus on the root cause of diseases. The media is busy pointing fingers at sick domestic or migratory birds while they ignore descriptions of their environment. If they did point their fingers at the conditions surrounding the sick birds, then certain corporate and financial interests would be very unhappy.

Farmers Understand that Hygiene Is the Major Reason Why Birds Get Sick

Most farmers are dubious about the emphasis being placed on "outdoor" birds, and with good reason. Charlie Walters grew up on a farm and has studied many aspects of agriculture, including economics. He is also concerned about the effects of chemicals on the environment, and so has spent a good deal of time studying organic farming practices. In order to share his knowledge of agriculture with farmers, Walters founded his own publication, *Acres USA*, in 1971. After meeting and interviewing several soil scientists, farm policy experts, economic thinkers, insect researchers, and philosophers of the land, in 1974 he decided to schedule an annual conference so that they could all meet to share their knowledge about agriculture.

At his conference, farmers meet to learn and share information about how to farm in a more natural way. The majority of the farmers who attend this conference farm organically—they use little to no chemicals or medications and raise their animals outdoors on pasture. Walters likes the term *eco-agriculture* as a way to describe a complete system of farming. If you want to imagine what that means, just think back about one hundred years before the corporations forced farmers into using the industrialized model.

Walters has his own reservations about the bird flu hysteria: "We are being told that bird flu could be such a pandemic that it will take us by the throat and throttle the life out of us—the truth of the matter is that it is just a sanitation problem and a nutrition problem. They are sick because they don't have enough nutritional support and they are not kept in good sanitary conditions and the people who work with these chickens will also get sick."[46]

This is just plain common sense to farmers who are using time-tested, sound agricultural practices to raise their chickens. They know that when the birds are outside basking in the sun and grazing on grass rich in minerals, they tend to be extremely healthy and resistant to diseases.

Farmers Care About the Quality of Your Food

If you have any doubt about the fact that our farmers have been manipulated and dealt with unfairly, all you need to do is look around the countryside and count just how many authentic farmers you can find. Knock on their doors and ask them if they're working for themselves or a corporation. The ones you will probably meet will likely be "serfs" to the corporations, not farmers. *The Big Chicken*, a documentary that aired on *60 Minutes* in December 1999, depicted the experience of modern chicken "farmers":

> A company owns their feed, the chickens and the fuel that they use to operate the facility. They have no control over their operation. No one can raise chickens independently anymore. A company can even make a farmer fail. [A] couple accused Perdue of sending them diseased chickens and feed that was damaged with too much moisture. The growers believed that this was a tactic used against them because of their efforts to organize a coalition of workers to protest corporate control.[47]

Charlie Walters describes the industrial poultry operators as "janitors" for the large corporations. Simply put, they have become slaves to a system that doesn't deserve to be called farming: "The birds are sick. If they don't get them slaughtered within 40 days, they wake up one morning and they are all dead in the house."[48] Walters can summarize the existence of CAFOs in one simple equation:

Big Business + Bad Science = CAFO

Don't be misled by advertising when a company says that they have the best chicken. Corporations make claims that they will "feed the world" with their genetic technologies and that they are a "sustainable" company—these claims couldn't be further from the truth. The primary responsibility of large corporations is to their shareholders, not to consumers. And, while it may be true that the corporations have literally taken over our food supply, it is the farmers who should really be responsible for feeding the world.

What would happen to the health of the chickens in a factory setting if they were eating what they were designed to eat? The industrial model forces these chickens to eat a synthetic concoction loaded with potential toxins and devoid of the many health-promoting phytonutrients and live insects that are a part of their normal diet. If the chickens were given any choice in the matter, they would certainly choose to graze outdoors before they would ever consider eating highly processed industry mush.

Corporations such as Tyson and Perdue rely heavily on the "all in, all out" industry model.[49] In other words, their primary focus is producing more animals in less time at the lowest cost, and selling as much as they possibly can, including by-products and dangerous waste. These corporations have subjected the planet to an environmental nightmare, and now we are all expected to tolerate what they've done. There are many hidden costs in food that are not paid at the checkout counter, but which ultimately will need to be reconciled.

You Can Make a Difference

We have paid a high price for cheap food, including the spread of diseases such as mad cow and the highly pathogenic bird flu. The trend in America has been to focus on convenience and price, at the expense of food quality. About 90 percent of the money that Americans spend on food goes to purchase processed food.[50] The primary beneficiaries of commercially processed foods are the companies that produce them—processing food increases the cost of the food as well as the profits for the manufacturer. Commercially processed foods are expensive in more ways than one—they cost more money, but they also jeopardize your health. You will find that when you return to a diet comprised of traditional whole foods, your food bill will probably go down and your health will improve. Seeking out healthier meat, chicken, pork, and dairy products from local pastured farms will also help improve your health and the health of your family.

Unfortunately, the typical consumer is not highly motivated to seek out high-quality foods, and will commonly seek the least expensive option in the store or, frequently, purchase similar food in the restaurant. Consumers blindly purchase their chicken meat and eggs not understanding the consequences of supporting the practice of factory farming. But if more people understood the detrimental side effects of industrial farming, they might invest a bit more time and energy and seek to purchase their food from healthier and more environmentally friendly sources.

Many savvy consumers are awakening to these issues. A number of colleges and universities, along with prominent employers such as America Online, food-service purveyors, restaurants, and even high schools, have either eliminated or reduced their use of eggs from caged hens. Colleges and universities that have instituted the policy include Yale, Tufts, Dartmouth, Vassar, and the University of Wisconsin. Another eighty schools made the switch when food service company Bon Appétit Management, which supplies their dining halls, went cage-free last October.[51] Cage-free chickens are still "indoor" birds, but they are probably a better choice than other commercial chickens or eggs, so at least it's a step in the right direction. The best choice is pastured or free-range chickens, or eggs from a local farm (it's important to make sure the chickens are outside so that they have access to pasture and are exposed to the sun).

You, too, can help reduce the power of the factory farms by simply not buying their food. The real solution to the problem is to start buying real food from real farms owned and operated by real farmers, instead of corporations and corporate serfs.

You don't have to give up eating chicken or eggs altogether. In local rural communities, pastured poultry producers raise their hens and broilers in a humane manner, allowing their birds to enjoy the benefits of a more natural environment. If you're unsure of their agricultural practices, you can simply drive out to their farm and see for yourself.

But if the media convinces you that only indoor grown chickens are safe to eat, then pastured poultry producers could potentially disappear. Companies like Tyson will stand to gain enormous profits if consumers only buy chicken produced in their bird jails.

Hopefully, this book will help as a resource and tool to enlighten individuals about the truth on this important topic. Public awareness could play a central role in the elimination of this problem. Up until the close of the twentieth century, vast corporate and government interests largely controlled the media. With the advent of the Internet, an open window of opportunity is present for the average person to make an incredible difference.

5

FOLLOW THE MONEY

How the Drug Companies Are Profiting from Fear

"All truth passes through three stages. First, it is ridiculed. Second, it is violently opposed. Third, it is accepted as being self-evident."

—ARTHUR SCHOPENHAUER, 1788–1860

As you continue to follow the money trail behind the bird flu alerts and warnings, you may be surprised to learn just how manipulated and deceived you've been over the last several decades. You may be astonished to find out how the media, government, and science have been influenced by significant corporate financial conflict of interests.

The sad reality is that the media, government, and universities have become unhealthily dependent upon corporate support. So the media reinforces their deception by feeding you stories and ads that will augment the corporate coffers and keep their shareholders happy. Politicians and bureaucrats support the corporate agendas to secure their reelection. Universities go out of their way to accommodate the corporations so that they can maintain their grant support funding.

As the bird flu panic sweeps around the world, many multinational corporations are orchestrating plans to take maximum advantage of this golden opportunity. There are many industries that stand to benefit from this hoax, not just the large chicken producers, but also major pharmaceutical companies and the biotech industry.

Biotech to the Rescue?

Many people fail to appreciate that the primary goal of multinational drug and biotech corporations is to increase the profits of their shareholders, NOT to serve humanity. Sure, their slick marketing would have you believe that they are altruistically motivated, but any objective, careful analysis will quickly cut through the deception. The design of the contemporary conventional health care system restricts the production of drugs to a few highly capitalized corporations, and their goal is profit and profit only.

If you want some clues about how contrived the bird flu disease profiteering is, just review the money sections of any of the mainstream media sources. Florida-based biotech company Viragen is just one biotech company among many that is racing to develop a genetically engineered vaccine for the bird flu. In a recent article in *CNN Money News*, Charles Rice, the CEO of Viragen, said that the company only focuses on blockbusters, or drugs with blockbuster potential. "There's no product that I could envision working on with less than $1 billion market value."[1] Rice projects that the biopharmaceutical (genetically engineered) drug market will generate an excess of $50 billion in sales by 2010.[2]

Viragen holds the worldwide exclusive license to commercialize Avian Transgenic Technology.[3] If their technology is successful, flocks of specially developed, genetically engineered chickens will produce eggs with high volumes of the target drug in the egg whites.[4]

Viragen believes that their technology holds significant promise for many new and powerful drugs that could be manufactured faster, cheaper, and in the virtually unlimited quantities needed to combat many serious and life-threatening diseases.[5]

Another potential financial boon for the biotech industry lies in the possible development of a chicken that is resistant to the H5N1 virus. In Britain, this project is already underway at Cambridge University. The team developing this H5N1 "transgenic chicken" is being led by Laurence Tiley, professor of Molecular Virology, and Helen Sang, PhD, of the Roslin Institute.[6] On October 29, 2005, Tiley told the *Times*, "Once we have regulatory approval, we believe it will only take between four and five years to breed enough chickens to replace the entire world [chicken] population."[7]

Perversion of Justice Allows Patents for Life Forms

For over two hundred years, the U.S. patent office refused to patent any life forms.[8] However, in an amazing perversion of justice, in 2001 the Monsanto corporation was successful in overturning the two-century-old tradition by appealing a case to the U.S. Supreme Court.[9] A 6–2 decision in Monsanto's favor upheld the patentability of genetically engineered plants and seeds. Before this decision, Congress had taken steps to keep plants in public hands, so that farmers could save some of their crop for the next planting season, even if they had inherited special characteristics developed by their seed supplier.

Since the 2001 case, however, the seed suppliers can control what is done with their genetically modified (GM) plants, and the farmers have no say in the matter.[10]

As it stands now, any organism, not just plant life, that has been genetically engineered is eligible for patenting and corporate profiteering.[11] So if anyone actuallly belives they need the "exclusive" H5N1 resistant chicken, or any other genetically engineered product in order to protect themselves from this nonexistent pandemic, then they will only be able to purchase it from the sole company that patents and produces it.

While corporations are busy "inventing" high-profit "solutions," they conveniently circumvent having to discuss the fact that a number of problems may be created by their bird jails. While this strategy will certainly increase their profits, it will only continue to exacerbate the problem. Genetically engineered products are fraught with controversy, primarily due to the fact that they have been produced and sold to consumers without adequate safety testing.

Most respected scientists advocate application of the precautionary principle ("if in doubt, leave it out") when it comes to the introduction of new technologies. Unfortunately, these concerns have been overridden by well-financed governmental lobbying efforts that have successfully subjugated concerns for your safety and the safety of your offspring to the maximization of corporate profits.

There are many examples of products that have been released on the market without proper scientific validation—pesticides, fluoride, margarine, aspartame, and others too innumerable to list here. Scientists who have not abandoned their integrity, as well as consumer advocacy groups, are fighting to have these products removed, but it is a complex and tortuous process once they have been initially approved by regulatory agencies.

Who Else is Benefiting From the Bird Flu Hoax?

On October 27, 2005, the Senate announced an emergency funding bill that would add $8 billion to the Department of Health and Human Services (HHS) budget to combat avian flu. As the late senator Everett Dirksen from Illinois was fond of saying when referring to Defense Department spending, "A billion dollars here and a billion dollars there, and soon it adds up to real money." Folks, this is an extraordinary amount of money; just imagine the number of ways those resources could be better spent.

Lawmakers said the bill would be able to fund of the soon-to-come White House flu preparedness plan.[12] The Senate plan included $3.3 billion to stockpile avian flu vaccines, and about $3 billion for antiviral drugs.[13] Just hours before the Senate made their announcement, Health and Human Services secretary Mike Leavitt awarded a $62.5 million contract to Emeryville, California-based Chiron Corp. to manufacture bird flu vaccine. And, in late August, federal health officials had also signed another $100 million vaccine contract with a competitor, Sanofi-Aventis of Paris.[14]

Senator Ted Stevens (R-Alaska), who leads the Senate Appropriations Committee, criticized the bill, saying, "That's just throwing money at the wall . . . It's political gimmickry."[15]

Shortly after the Senate announcement, on November 1, 2005, President George W. Bush announced the "Pandemic Influenza Strategic Plan."[16] Despite the lack of any evidence for a bird flu pandemic, the president ordered Congress to approve $7.1 billion in emergency funding to prepare for one. The following is a list of how President Bush plans to allocate the money:

- $2.8 billion to accelerate development of cell-culture technology

- $1.5 billion for the Department of Health and Human Services to purchase influenza vaccines

- $1.0 billion to stockpile antiviral medication

- $600 million to develop new antiflu drugs and better annual vaccines

- $251 million to detect and contain outbreaks before they spread around the world

- $100 million for states to make plans on how to respond to an outbreak

- $56 million to test poultry and wild birds for H5N1

- $1.1 billion for other spending[17]

The U.S. government intends to buy 75 million doses of antiviral drugs (Tamiflu) in order to combat any outbreak of pandemic flu.[18] Several other countries have also ordered significant amounts of this drug. In March of 2005, the UK ordered 14.5 million courses of Tamiflu, which will only partially supply its 56 million citizens.[19, 20] Germany has ordered 6 million doses of Tamiflu, and France, New Zealand, and Norway all plan to purchase enough to treat 20–25 percent of their populations.[21] And in Canada, the government has stockpiled 35 million doses of Tamiflu.[22]

As you will soon read, there is virtually no evidence that Tamiflu would work against a highly infectious virus. But Swiss-U.S. pharmaceutical giant Roche Holdings of Basle will still get paid $1 billion dollars by the U.S. government for Tamiflu stockpiles, all due to the concern generated by the bird flu hoax.

> **Swiss-U.S. pharmaceutical giant Roche Holdings of Basle will still get paid $1 billion dollars by the U.S. government for Tamiflu stockpiles, all due to the concern generated by the bird flu hoax.**

It's likely you even know a few people who have already pressured their doctor into giving them a prescription, and have already rushed off to the local pharmacy to secure their doses for themselves and their family. Unfortunately, this practice is facilitated by third-party insurance carriers that pay the bulk of exorbitant fees for these expensive drugs, disguising their ultimate price. The typical consumer would not rush to purchase these expensive drug solutions unless they were covered by an insurance policy.

While you, your friends, and your family won't benefit from Tamiflu, there are others that will. The U.S. secretary of defense Donald Rumsfeld was on the board of Gilead Sciences, the company that developed Tamiflu, between 1988 and 2001, and was chairman starting in 1997.[23] When he left to join the Bush administration, he retained a large shareholding.

When Donald Rumsfeld left the board of Gilead, its stock price was sitting at around $7.00 per share. But when Bush announced his pandemic plan, the stock price skyrocketed to over $50.00 per share.[24] Rumsfeld then made more than $5 million from selling shares in the firm, and he retains shares worth $25 million or more.[25] Before concerns about bird flu began, the company was taking losses. But over the past two years, Tamiflu sales nearly quadrupled, and then nearly quadrupled again.[26]

> **Donald Rumsfeld made more than $5 million from selling shares in the firm, and he retains shares worth $25 million or more.**

Tamiflu—Great For Drug Company Profits and Nearly Worthless for Bird Flu

Earlier flu drugs like amantadine and rimantadine proved highly ineffective for the treatment of bird flu, so researchers have sought newer (and more expensive) solutions.[27] Tamiflu was introduced on the market in 1999, and Roche Pharmaceuticals says that 33 million people in roughly eighty countries have now used the drug.[28] Tamiflu's generic name is *oseltamivir*, and it was developed from the unusual fruit of a small oriental tree, the star anise. Roche recently announced that by the end of 2006, it would increase production of Tamiflu to 400 million treatments.[29] More than sixty-five countries have now ordered Tamiflu with the intention of stockpiling it in preparation for a bird flu pandemic.[30]

Tamiflu is considered a "patient friendly" drug because it can be taken orally, rather than by injection like some of the earlier flu drugs, such as Relenza. Many are confused and believe that Tamiflu is a vaccine, but it is not; it's an antiviral drug.

With all the people using the drug, you would think it must be an incredibly effective solution for the flu. But nothing could be further from the truth. While the drug does have some effect on the flu, the ONLY benefit the manufacturers were able to prove is that it shortens the symptoms of seasonal flu by one day.

Yes, you read that correctly. One day. It reduces, not eliminates, your flu symptoms by about twenty-four hours. How many people would be willing to pay the $100+ price for this drug if they knew this?

On the Web site www.tamiflu.com, it is claimed that in the "Last flu season, doctors wrote more prescriptions for Tamiflu than any other flu treatment. Tamiflu attacks the influenza virus and stops it from spreading inside your body." The Tamiflu Web site goes on to say that "in adult treatment studies, flu patients who took Tamiflu felt better 1.3 days faster (30 percent) than flu patients who did not take Tamiflu."[31]

Dr. Shiv Chopra, veterinarian and microbiologist, has evaluated drugs for humans and animals. He says that Tamiflu would not be effective against a bird flu epidemic and adds that, it isn't particularly effective against seasonal flu either.[32]

It is also important to note that the symptom reduction has

ONLY been proven for seasonal flu, and NOT for the bird flu. Tamiflu was designed to treat the run-of-the-mill conventional flu. The drug was never intended to be used for the bird flu, but it has been conveniently revectored into the "drug of choice" for "protection" against and treatment of a potential bird flu pandemic.

> **Tamiflu was designed to treat the run-of-the-mill conventional flu. The drug was never intended to be used for the bird flu.**

As of June 2006, there were no published studies on the use of Tamiflu for the bird flu. In Dr. Sherry Tenpenny's recent book *Fowl! Bird Flu: It's Not What You Think*, she revealed some interesting unpublished work on Tamiflu's remarkable ineffectiveness against avian influenza.[33] Dr. Tenpenny is an outspoken critic of conventional medicine who is Board Certified in Emergency Medicine and Osteopathic Manipulative Medicine.

To make her points a bit clearer, you should first know that influenza viruses have two important protein antigens that are on the surface. One is called heamagglutinin (H) and the other is the enzyme neuraminidase (N), which plays an important role in the effective spread of the virus.[34] Tamiflu is technically classified as a neuraminidase inhibitor, and works by blocking the (N) antigen of influenza viruses.[35] Tamiflu, and drugs like it, have absolutely no effect on other viruses that cause influenza-like illnesses.

Here's what Dr. Tenpenny uncovered regarding Tamiflu:

> In laboratory tests designed to evaluate Tamiflu's ability to inhibit the N1 neuraminidase, Tamiflu failed dismally. In order for it to work, eight to twelve times the recommended dose of the drug was needed to achieve the same level of inhibition in other subtypes.[36]

But wait—it gets even better:

> When Tamiflu was actually tested specifically against H5N1 strains of the virus from Vietnam and Thailand, an additional three-fold increase in the dose was required to stop its activities, meaning almost 30 times more Tamiflu would be needed to stop the infectivity of H5N1 than other form of influenza virus.[37]

That much Tamiflu would cost nearly $3,000. And for that price, you could achieve the wonderful benefit of reducing, not eliminating, your symptoms by a mere twenty-four hours.

However, two important factors are excluded from this analysis: drug resistance and side effects. There has already been careful documentation of resistance to Tamiflu when it has been used to treat bird flu.[38, 39, 40]

Dr. Moscana, a flu expert at Weill Cornell Medical College in New York City, recently conducted a comprehensive review of this topic that was published in the *New England Journal of Medicine*.[41] The full text of this excellent article is available at no charge online on the *Journal*'s Web site .[42] Dr. Moscana reported that Tamiflu might not be as effective in treating the bird flu virus as had been anticipated; even after being given Tamiflu, four out of eight H5N1 infected Vietnamese patients died.[43] Dr. Moscana called the deaths frightening.[44]

In early 2006, a review published in the *Lancet* medical journal found no evidence that Tamiflu would be effective in the event of a human bird flu pandemic.[45, 46] Tom Jefferson, the author of the review, noted that Tamiflu did not reduce mortality from bird flu in the few victims who had taken the drug, and added that "relying on a single solution is suicidal."[47]

After following World Health Organization protocols in treating forty-one victims of the H5N1 bird flu virus, Dr. Nguyen Tuong

Van, who runs the intensive care unit of the Center for Tropical Diseases in Hanoi, Vietnam, concluded that Tamiflu is "useless."[48] According to Van, Tamiflu had no effect on the disease. The WHO also notes that Tamiflu has not been "widely successful in human patients."[49]

A 2004 Japanese study found that 18 percent of children with an Influenza A (H3N2) virus infection who had been treated with Tamiflu developed resistance to the drug.[50] Additional research in Japanese children found that treated viruses could be 300-fold to 1,000-fold more resistant than non-Tamiflu treated viruses.[51]

Tamiflu may actually influence the mutation of more dangerous and aggressive forms of the virus. This has led many respectable scientists to question the wisdom of using drugs as a first line of defense in any bird flu epidemic, as these drugs could actually cause the very pandemic that government officials and health experts are seeking to avoid.[52]

The Potential Side Effects of Tamiflu

Most of the research on Tamiflu comes from Japan, because the drug is used far more commonly there than in most other countries. Nearly 25 million prescriptions for Tamiflu were filled in Japan in 2005, while there were only one-fifth that number of prescriptions filled in the United States during the same period. Nearly 11 million children were given Tamiflu in Japan in 2005, while less than 1 million children received the drug in the United States This is in part because it was only approved for pediatric use in the U.S. in March of 2004.

In November 2005, after a group of Japanese children had taken Tamiflu to treat seasonal flu, twelve died, and thirty-two more reportedly experienced neuropsychiatric "incidents," including seizures, loss of consciousness, and delirium.[53,54] The Japanese Health

Ministry has added neurological and psychological disorders to the list of possible adverse effects associated with Tamiflu. In the United States, however, the FDA immediately dismissed these concerns,[55] although they did add a warning to Tamiflu's Product Information—stating that taking Tamiflu was associated with rashes.[56]

Side Effects of Tamiflu— Other Possible Dangers of Using It

The FDA's Web site lists these symptoms as possible side effects associated with taking Tamiflu:

- Nausea
- Vomiting
- Diarrhea
- Bronchitis
- Stomach pain
- Dizziness or
- Headache[57]

Drugs.com also lists a variety of other possible side effects, which include:

- Wheezing
- Abdominal cramps
- Arm, back, chest, or jaw pain
- Facial swelling
- Irregular heartbeat and
- Fever[58]

Other possible side effects could include:

- Insomnia

- Anemia

- Pneumonia

- Dermatitis

- Eczema

- Stevens-Johnson-Syndrome

- Anaphylaxis

- Toxic epidermal necrolysis

- Abnormal liver function

- Cardiac arrhythmia

- Seizure

- Confusion or

- Aggravation of diabetes[59]

Various cases of psychological disorders, such as delerium and hallucinations, have been associated with taking Tamiflu, some severe enough to result in deaths.[60]

According to German virologist and molecular biologist Dr. Stephan Lanka:

> Those side effects which are noted on the instruction slips accompanying packages of Tamiflu are *almost identical to the symptoms* of a serious influenza [emphasis added]. Thus, on a large scale, medicines are now being stored which cause precisely the same symptoms as those which appear in an actual so-called influenza. If Tamiflu is administered to sick persons, then this is

likely to cause far more serious symptoms than those of a serious influenza.

If a pandemic is stated to exist, then many people will take this medicine at the same time. In that case we will actually have unequivocal symptoms of a Tamiflu epidemic. Then *deaths caused by Tamiflu are to be expected*, and this will then be presented as evidence of the dangerous nature of the bird flu and evidence of how anxious the state is that people should be in good health [emphasis added].[61]

Bird Flu Vaccine—Another Expensive False Hope Solution

The alternative to Tamiflu most commonly proposed has been the development of a vaccine that protects against the H5N1 virus. Sanofi Pasteur, Chiron, Baxter, PowerMed and NIAID are only a few examples of companies and organizations performing trial studies on vaccines intended to fight the highly pathogenic bird flu—rest assured there will be more. The federal government has allocated over $3.3 billion dollars to develop a vaccine to fight the bird flu, so there is plenty of money to go around. Some of the companies that have received this money are trying to hasten the process of making vaccines.

Like Tamiflu, however, the vaccine solution is based on fantasy. Both are clever schemes to transfer funds to the pharmaceutical industry for developing solutions to a problem that is virtually assured never to materialize; and even if it did materialize, the vaccine solution also has little to no chance of success, based on the long-standing history of the conventional flu vaccine.

Vaccines might be more effective than Tamiful (although, as you will see, still too unsafe to be worth the risk), but it's simply impossible to develop one that would be effective against bird flu on any reasonable timescale. Viruses change over time, and by the time a vaccine is developed and manufactured, it will probably no longer work.[62]

According to Dr. Anthony Fauci, immunologist and the head of the National Institute of Allergy and Infectious Diseases (NIAID), as of March 2, 2006, "Right now, the vaccine that we've made is based on a 2004 strain that we isolated from a Vietnamese patient. We call that a pre-pandemic vaccine. So it is likely that that vaccine, if the virus changes, is not going to be as efficient as you would want it to be against the strain that ultimately does become the real problem."[63]

On November 14, 2005, *Wired* magazine reported that ". . . it will take at least five years to create enough manufacturing capacity to reach that goal [of making enough vaccine for every American]. Then it will take another eight months to create a new vaccine that combats the specific strain that would be killing people. In other words, *it would be 2011 at the earliest before every American could be vaccinated against a bird flu pandemic.*"[64, 65] The Congressional Budget Office also estimated that 2011 would be the earliest the vaccine manufacturers could produce enough vaccine.[66]

Please remember, even if enough vaccine could be manufactured in time, the effectiveness of such a plan is based on two very large assumptions: first, that the vaccine would work, and second, that there would be minimal side effects. Considering the history of the flu vaccine, such as its disastrous use during the swine flu scare, I have serious reservations about any possibility of an effective and safe bird flu vaccine.

I rarely gamble, and can honestly say I have been in Vegas many times and have never even placed any bets or played any slots. However, I believe that an attempt to produce a safe, effective bird flu vaccine is as close to a guaranteed failure as it comes, and I would seriously consider betting very heavily against its success.

New Vaccine Legislation May Abolish
Your Seventh Amendment Rights

In October 2005, when the "Biodefense and Pandemic Vaccine and Drug Development Act of 2005" (S. 1873) passed out of the U.S. Senate Health, Education, Labor, and Pensions (HELP) Committee, the National Vaccine Information Center (NVIC) called the proposed bill, "a drug company stockholder's dream and a consumer's worst nightmare."[67]

This bill, spurred by bird flu fears, will broadly eliminate corporate liability for vaccines and drugs. The purported intent of the bill is "to prepare and strengthen the biodefenses of the United States against deliberate, accidental and natural outbreaks of illness, and for other purposes,"[68] but it is a cleverly disguised tool of the pharmaceutical industry to legally confiscate even more wealth and then insulate themselves from any potential future liability from the inevitable side effects that will be produced by the expensive vaccines they will push on the public.

The proposed legislation, nicknamed "Bioshield II," is being pushed rapidly through Congress without time for voters to contact their elected representatives. If this bill passes, it will strip Americans of their constitutional right to a trial by jury if they are harmed by a drug or vaccine, even one that may be forced upon them by the government if federal officials declare a public health emergency.

This bill passed through the Senate one day after it was introduced, and just days before President George W. Bush announced his "Pandemic Influenza Strategic Plan."

The bill establishes the Biomedical Advanced Research and Development Agency (BARDA) as the single point of authority within the government for research and development of drugs and vaccines in response to bioterrorism and natural disease outbreaks. BARDA will operate secretly, exempt from the Freedom of Information Act and the Federal Advisory Committee Act, ensuring that no evidence of injuries or deaths caused by drugs and vaccines labeled as "countermeasures" will ever become public.

This proposed legislation is an unconstitutional attempt by some in Congress to provide a taxpayer-funded subsidy to pharmaceutical companies for drugs and vaccines that the government can then mandate that the public must receive. It will absolve the manufacturers of the vaccine, who will earn all the profits, from having any responsibility for injuries and deaths that occur as a result of their flawed product.

As Barbara Loe Fisher, president of NVIC, puts it, "It is a sad day for this nation when Congress is frightened and bullied into allowing one profit making industry to destroy the seventh Amendment to the Constitution guaranteeing citizens their day in court in front of a jury of their peers."[69]

An NVIC press release emphasizes that

> [i]f the . . . bill passes, all economic incentives to insure mandated vaccines are safe will be removed and the American people are facing a future where government can force them to take poorly regulated experimental drugs and vaccines labeled as "countermeasures" or go to jail. The only recourse for citizens will be to strike down mandatory vaccination laws so vaccines will be subject to the law of supply and demand in the marketplace. The health care consumer's cry will be: No liability? No mandates.[70]

On June 30, 2006, the FDA "Final Rule" went into effect. Similar to Bioshield II, it established that consumers can no longer sue drug companies for the harm caused by any FDA-approved drug, even if the drug's manufacturer intentionally misled the FDA by hiding or fabricating clinical trial data.[71]

Currently, there are an unprecedented number of lawsuits against the medical community. It has been estimated that the total number of deaths caused by conventional medicine is an astounding 783,936 per year.[72] Protecting the pharmaceutical industry is the last thing the government needs to be doing.

The cozy relationship between the government and the pharmaceutical companies regarding the bird flu vaccine is once again reminiscent of the days of the swine flu scare. During that period, prominent vaccine researcher Dr. J. Anthony Morris (formerly of HEW and director of the Virus Bureau at the FDA) was fired after he criticized the swine flu vaccine. He pointed out that there could be no authentic swine flu vaccine because there had never been any human cases of swine flu on which they could test it.[73] He publicly announced, "At no point were the swine flu vaccines effective."[74]

Morris hired prominent Washington lawyer Jim Turner to defend his case. Turner recounts Dr. Morris's criticisms of vaccine regulation: "From top to bottom vaccine regulation was laced with bad thinking, bad policy, bad implementation, and lots of peoples' lives were put at risk because of the way vaccine policy was being done."[75]

At the time of the swine flu scare, Turner recalls that officials were so desperate to find cases of the swine flu in the United States they tried to label an outbreak of Legionnaire's disease, which occurred in Philadelphia, as being the swine flu. Over the eight-year legal battle, Turner concluded that "one of the primary if not the primary reason for the existence of these programs and of these people and these efforts is to make money for companies."[76]

Dr. Barbara Law, chief of vaccine safety for the Public Health Agency of Canada, reminds us that "the [swine flu] vaccine killed more people than the flu itself, so fear of a similar result hangs over current plans for rushed mass vaccinations against bird flu."[77]

Dr. Barbara Law, chief of vaccine safety for the Public Health Agency of Canada, reminds us that "the [swine flu] vaccine killed more people than the flu itself, so fear of a similar result hangs over current plans for rushed mass vaccinations against bird flu."

By January of 1977, more than 500 cases of the crippling Guillain-Barré Syndrome had been reported, with, as you will recall, 25 deaths.[78] Understandably, the deaths and injuries caused by the swine flu vaccine sparked a wave of lawsuits.[79] The U.S. government ended up paying claimants around $90 million.[80]

This might explain why Bush is pushing to protect drug companies against anticipated lawsuits this time around; since the bird flu hoax is very similar to the swine flu debacle, it is likely to yield the same results.

Do Vaccines Prevent
or Actually Cause Disease?

One of the great modern-day myths is that the government vaccination programs are safe and effective. The fact of the matter is, vaccines are not at all the safe, effective cure-all that they have been promoted to be by the drug companies and conventional medical system. As you will see in the charts below, the greatest decline in the U.S. death rate actually occurred in the first half of the twentieth century, before the "benefits" of nearly all of the modern vaccines were available. American mortality rates declined the most after sanitation projects reduced the spread of disease in the U.S. water supply.

Treatments of drinking water began in the early 1900s and became widespread public health practices, decreasing the incidence of many diseases.[81] From the 1930s through the 1950s, further progress in disease prevention was attributed to:

- Sewage disposal
- Water treatment
- Food safety
- Organized solid waste disposal[82]
- Public education about hygienic practices (e.g., foodhandling and handwashing)
- Improvements in housing (reduced crowding).

Harold Buttram, MD, recently wrote that "from 1911 to 1935 the four leading causes of childhood deaths from infectious diseases in the U.S. were diphtheria, pertussis (whooping cough), scarlet fever and measles. However, by 1945 the combined death rates from these causes had declined by 95 percent, before the implementation of mass immunization programs."[83] Remember the important point—

> **Death rates for almost all vaccine-"preventable" diseases decreased significantly before the development, licensing, and universal use of that vaccine.**

National efforts to promote vaccine use among all children began with the introduction of the polio vaccine in 1955. So, while vaccines for whooping cough, tetanus, and tuberculosis were all developed in the 1920s, they were not widely used in the United States until after deaths from the diseases had already dropped to negligible amounts.[84] The first measles vaccine wasn't licensed until 1963, when deaths from the disease had already dropped from 14.1 per 100,000 to just 0.2.

You'll see an apparent drop in diphtheria deaths on the charts after the vaccine was introduced, but the vaccine was not actually promoted among children until the late 1940s, after the death rate had already dropped from 40.3 per 100,000 down to 0.9. And as for the flu, in 1900 it caused 202.2 deaths per 100,000. During the great influenza pandemic of 1918, that number shot up to 588.5. By the time the flu vaccine was licensed in 1945, it had already dropped to 51.6 and was descending rapidly.[85]

Infectious Disease Mortality Rates

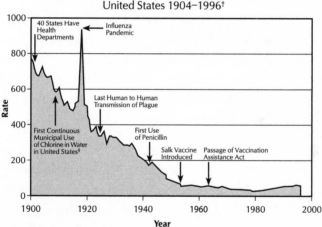

Crude Death Rate* for Infectious Diseases[86]
United States 1904–1996[†]

*Per 100,000 population per year.
[†]Adapted from Armstrong GL, Conn LA, Pinner RW. Trends in infectious disease mortlity in the United States during the 20th century. JAMA 1999:281;61–6.
[§]American Water Works Association. Water chlorination principles and practices: AWAA manual M20. Denver, Colorado: American Water Works Association, 1973

United States Mortality Rates

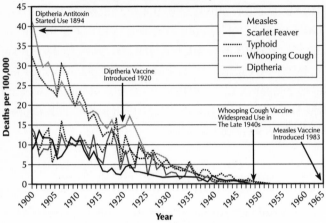

References: Vital Statistics of the United States 1937, 1938, 1943,1944, 1944, 1960, 1967, 1976, 1987, 1992; Historical Statistics of the United States – Colonial Times to 1970 Part 1

Used with permission from www.healthsentinel.com

What Vaccines Really Prevent

Contrary to what you have been led to believe for most of your life, vaccines really impair your ability to achieve high-level health. Many critics of vaccines argue that they cause more harm than good. Although mortality rates dropped before the development of vaccines, the rates of many chronic illnesses, such as cancer, have actually increased dramatically since their introduction.[87]

While the above probably sounds like medical heresy if you are new to natural medicine, I implore you to take a few deep breaths, calm yourself, and carefully and objectively examine the evidence. Avoid the temptation to dismiss this as a bunch of rubbish because experts you trust say otherwise.

The vaccine issue is one of the most controversial topics in medicine, and typically one of the last positions a conventionally trained physician will relinquish once they carefully study the issue.

I know that was true for me, and it took me many years to change my views of Dr. Robert Mendelsohn, one of the major pioneers in this area.[88]

Dr. Mendelsohn wrote numerous books, articles, and studies explaining that some of the greatest causes of childhood diseases were actually the dangerous and ineffective vaccines used in an attempt to prevent them.[89] Like most physicians, I viewed him as a dangerous, ignorant quack who clearly did not understand what he was talking about, and whose views were putting innocent children at risk. However, I gradually learned more about the risks of vaccines and began to see hundreds of brain-injured children in my practice—children who had been damaged by vaccines. My views changed quite dramatically.

I now regret never having met Dr. Mendelsohn, especially since we both worked out of the University of Illinois, where I went to school. Dr. Mendelsohn was a brave man who dared to tell the truth, and stood up to the conventional system in order to protect kids from the harm that vaccines were causing.

So I urge you to not make the same mistake I did twenty years ago and quickly dismiss this issue because it conflicts with what you were taught. For your sake and, more importantly, for the sake of your children, please examine this issue very carefully before you pass judgment on it.

Doctors Against Vaccines

In researching his book *Murder by Injection*, Eustace Mullins uncovered a long history of vaccine dissenters. One physician, Dr. Henry R. Bybee, publicly stated, "My honest opinion is that vaccine is the cause of more disease and suffering than anything I could name. I believe that such diseases as cancer, syphilis, cold sores and many other disease conditions are the direct results of vaccination. Yet, in the state of Virginia, and many other states, parents are compelled to submit their children to this procedure while the medical profession not only receives its pay for this service, but also makes splendid and prospective patients for the future."[90]

Dr. Herbert Snow, senior surgeon at the Cancer Hospital of London, voiced his concern: "In recent years many men and women in the prime of life have dropped dead suddenly . . . I am convinced that some eighty percent of these deaths are caused by the inoculation or vaccination they have undergone. They are well known to cause grave and permanent disease of the heart."[91]

Another practitioner, Dr. W. B. Clarke, notes that "cancer was practically unknown until compulsory vaccination . . . began to be introduced. I have had to deal with at least two hundred cases of cancer, and I never saw a case of cancer in an unvaccinated person."[92]

In his book, Mullins cites a quote that Jonas Salk, developer of the polio vaccine, cowrote with his son, Dr. Darrell Salk. They warned us over forty years ago that "live virus vaccines against influenza or poliomyelitis may in each instance produce the disease it intended to prevent—the live virus against measles and mumps may produce such side effects as encephalitis (brain damage)."[93]

According to Mullins, some medical historians believe that the 1918 flu pandemic was actually a disease-and-reaction cocktail caused by the widespread use of typhoid, smallpox and other vaccines when, during WWI, such vaccinations were made compulsory for all servicemen.[94] Mullins found information in the *Boston Herald* reporting that forty-seven soldiers had been killed by vaccinations in one month.[95]

Dr. J. M. Peebles of San Francisco, a well-known medical practitioner, has also written a book on vaccine, in which he says,

"The vaccination practice, pushed to the front on all occasions by the medical profession through political connivance made compulsory by the state, has not only become the chief menace and the greatest danger to the health of the rising generation, but likewise the crowning outrage upon the personal liberties of the American citizen; compulsory vaccination, poisoning the crimson currents of the human system with brute-extracted lymph under the strange infatuation that it would prevent smallpox, was one of the darkest blots that disfigured the last century."[96]

All is Not Lost—There Is Hope

The threat of the bird flu has been a financial boon for the pharmaceutical industry, and the federal government has cooperated and facilitated their efforts to increase their revenues from this perceived threat with their ineffective and potentially dangerous drugs and vaccines.

You may be asking yourself, at this point, what you can do. Even if the bird flu is not actually a threat, other infectious diseases genuinely do kill thousands each year. If drugs and vaccines don't work and can even be deadly, and the very food you buy in the stores is toxic and dangerous, what can you do to keep yourself safe?

One of the best ways to protect yourself is by making informed diet and lifestyle changes that incorporate natural lifestyle principles. There are a large number of experts you can review; however, if you find this area confusing and are looking for guidance you can find many consistent and specific recommendations on my Web site at Mercola.com. You can boost your immune system and prevent both infectious and chronic diseases with simple, practical choices made on a daily basis. Ignore the Band-Aid solutions offered by federal government and the pharmaceutical industry and instead take proactive measures to improve your health.

6

NATURAL CURES

Improving Your Immune System
to Protect Yourself from the Bird Flu

The mainstream media would have you believe that there are only a few things you can do to ward off the bird flu. If you follow their advice, then you may have already started washing your hands more often. Perhaps you've also purchased a case of face masks, or stocked up on Tamiflu.

The panic and paranoia surrounding the bird flu is sufficient to negatively influence your immune system and make you sick. So if you have been distressed about this topic, the first step is to take a few deep breaths, calm down, and relax so that you can make the proper decisions for you and your family's health.

Prevention is Your Best Bet

If you are interested in natural health, you may be hearing about several different alternative "remedies" for either the bird flu or the regular seasonal flu. Some Web sites tout colloidal silver, while others may recommend Echinacea or other herbal remedies. There are, in fact, a number of things you can do that will help you to restore or build your immune system. But the answers are much less complicated than you have typically been led to believe.

You shouldn't need the threat of a pandemic to shock you into improving your diet and lifestyle, but for some, that may be exactly what it takes. And if you do improve your health habits, chances are you won't "catch" the flu at all.

> You shouldn't need the threat of a pandemic to shock you into improving your diet and lifestyle, but for some, that may be exactly what it takes. And if you do improve your health habits, chances are you won't "catch" the flu at all.

Band-Aid Solutions Are
Prescriptions for Disaster

Now, let's make it clear at the outset that I have nothing against Band-Aids. In fact, I am very grateful that they exist, both literally and metaphorically. Sometimes you simply don't have a choice, and you must rely on a temporary fix to get you out of a jam. However, when that temporary fix becomes the primary method used to address the problem at hand, it's simply asking for trouble.

Unfortunately, that is precisely what conventional medical care has evolved into over the last hundred years. Researchers have been able to uncover some important relationships between lifestyle and disease, but this limited knowledge has evolved into a professional arrogance that has played a major role in the explosion of chronic degenerative diseases in the twentieth century.

In 1912, when Dr. Casimir Funk discovered the nutritional link between vitamin B1 and the disease beriberi, he didn't intend to open the floodgates for a new multibillion dollar vitamin industry.

He had originally set out to discover why there was an outbreak of beriberi (a nervous system disorder) in Asia. He suspected that it had something to do with the fact that Asians had shifted from a diet based on whole grain brown rice to white (dehulled) rice, a simple starch. He was right; according to William Dufty, author of the book *Sugar Blues*, "After the introduction of refined white sugar and white polished rice on Japanese battleships, beriberi began plaguing the sailors . . ."[1]

After months of studying rice hulls, Funk discovered a vital substance that he believed was missing from white rice: the nutrient vitamin B1, also called thiamine. He concluded that the outbreak of beriberi in Asia was caused by a deficiency in this vitamin.

Funk intended that his research be used to help reintroduce brown rice back into the Asian diet. But his discovery led to a very different result. When Dr. Robert R. Williams published the chemical formula of vitamin B1 in the 1930s, scientists, doctors and investors understood the implications of being able to create this new vitamin synthetically in a lab. They realized that it could be used to "treat" nutritional disorders such as beriberi.

Some marketing geniuses realized that they couldn't make money convincing people to eat brown rice, but they could reap major financial rewards by selling synthetic vitamin B1. Funk made valiant efforts to stop the industry from exploiting his discovery, but it was too late. He argued, "What would be the use of preparing all our foods artificially as long as nature is producing her own foods in sufficient abundance . . . It would be folly even to think of turning ourselves into domestic manufacturers and consumers of self-made food as long as nature gives us enough."[2]

If you truly want to achieve optimal health—and give your body the best chance possible to fight off invaders like the bird flu—you simply cannot rely on Band-Aid solutions like supplements and drugs to treat your symptoms. They in no way, shape, or form address the underlying cause of your health challenges, but merely serve as a temporary and potentially dangerous respite from your symptoms. To maintain ideal health, it is vital to take steps to adjust your diet and lifestyle in ways that address the roots of the problem, rather than simply suppressing symptoms with potentially toxic Band-Aids.

Sugar and Most Grains Can Negatively Affect Your Immune System

One of the most important changes you can make to keep yourself from becoming ill is to avoid sugar. Sugar decreases the function of many aspects of your immune system almost immediately, and a strong immune system is an important key to fighting off viruses and other illnesses, including the flu.

It is especially imperative to avoid sugar if you feel you are struggling with a current infection. However, excluding sugar from your diet long term will do wonders for your health and help make your immune system stronger, which will make it more difficult for the flu to take hold in the first place.

Other simple carbohydrates, such as grains and potatoes, should also be avoided, for much the same reasons. Yes, this even includes grains commonly perceived as "healthy," like organic whole wheat, millet, quinoa, or amaranth. Even though these grains are far healthier than their highly processed equivalents, they are very different from vegetable carbohydrates and break down into sugar relatively quickly. This rapid breakdown raises insulin levels, which will impair your immune response.

For ages, humans existed on a diet of animals and gathered vegetation. It was only with the advent of agriculture a mere ten thousand years ago that humans began ingesting large amounts of refined sugars and starchy grains into their diets. But 99.99 percent of your genes were present before the advent of agriculture; in biological terms, your body still retains many characteristic of your ancient hunter-gatherer ancestors.

The shift to agriculture produced indisputable gains; modern civilization stems from this development. But the transition from a primarily meat and vegetable diet to one high in cereals has resulted in a reduction in lifespan and stature, increases in infant mortality and infectious disease, and a higher incidence of nutritional deficiencies.[3] Some doctors fear that the nutritional and health standards have deteriorated so much that the current generation of children will not live as long as their parents.[4]

Contemporary humans did not suddenly evolve mechanisms to successfully incorporate starch- and sugar-rich foods into their diet. Your body is not designed to consume so much bread, cereal, pasta, corn (which is a grain), rice, and potatoes, not to mention the concentrated sugars in most highly processed junk foods. Eating them in large quantities can have very serious negative consequences to your health.

Sixty-five percent of Americans are overweight, and 27 percent are clinically obese. But these are just numbers, and probably numbers you have been exposed to before. What is really startling about these numbers is the rate at which they have been increasing. To see a powerful visual illustration of the rapid increase in obesity on a state by state basis, I encourage you go to www.GreatBirdFluHoax.com/fat.

It is no coincidence that this increase in obesity is occurring in a nation addicted to sesame seed buns for their hamburgers, with a side of French fries and a Coke. It is not the fat in the foods we eat but, far more, the excess carbohydrates from our starch- and sugar-loaded diet that is making people fat and unhealthy, and leading to epidemic levels of a host of diseases such as diabetes. Last year the number one source of calories in America shifted from white bread to the sugar in regular sodas.[5] Clearly, the majority of American calories are from junk food.

You need a certain amount of carbohydrates in your diet, of

course, but your body's storage capacity for carbohydrates is actually quite limited, and excesses are converted via insulin into fat, and stored in your adipose, or fatty, tissue. Meals or snacks high in carbohydrates generate a rapid rise in blood glucose. To adjust for this rise, your pancreas secretes the hormone insulin into your bloodstream, which lowers your blood sugar level. Insulin, though, is essentially a storage hormone, designed to store the excess calories from carbohydrates in the form of fat.

Even worse, high insulin levels suppress two other important hormones—glucagons and growth hormones—that are responsible for burning fat and sugar and promoting muscle development, respectively. So insulin from excess carbohydrates promotes fat and then wards off your body's ability to lose that fat.

Excess weight and obesity lead to heart disease and a wide variety of other chronic diseases. Grains and sugars also contribute to allergies by suppressing the immune system, are responsible for a host of digestive disorders, and contribute to depression. But the ill effect of grains and sugars does not end there.

If you are experiencing any of the following symptoms, chances are very good that the excess carbohydrates in your body are, in part or whole, to blame:

- Excess weight
- Fatigue and frequent sleepiness
- Depression
- Brain fogginess
- Bloating
- Low blood sugar
- High blood pressure
- High triglycerides

So, during any acute infection, it is wise to avoid grains, even healthier ones, until you recover your health. However, continuing this grain exclusion even when you are well would likely benefit over 75 percent of the population, because in addition to having adverse effects on your immune response, elevated insulin levels are also factors in the following common health problems:

- Obesity

- Cancer

- Heart Disease

- Diabetes

I have also used a system called Metabolic Typing that assesses one's individual biochemical differences to help predict a person's ideal balance of proteins, carbs, and fats. It has been nothing less than extraordinary in my practice, and if you are interested in learning more about this you can go to: www.GreatBirdFluHoax.com/mt.

Exercise Is More Potent Than Most Drugs

Exercise also helps to improve your immune system by normalizing insulin levels. In addition, when you exercise, you increase your circulation and your blood flow throughout your body. The components of your immune system are therefore also better circulated, which means your immune system has a better chance of finding an illness before it has a chance to spread. In a sense, exercising helps your immune system to be more efficient in weeding out and acting upon viruses and diseases.

Choose an exercise that you enjoy doing. Keep experimenting until you find the exercise that you like. It could be tennis, golf, running, yoga, walking—whatever you enjoy.

Here are some key points to remember when exercising:

Listen to your body. If exercise worsens your symptoms, modify your program or, if need be, stop. As your energy and health improve, you will be able to tolerate larger amounts of aerobic exercise. It can help to hire a personal trainer who can guide you through the specifics of a good exercise program.

Be consistent. You need at least thirty minutes of exercise a day to experience any benefits. Major studies have shown that sixty minutes a day is actually best. According to Dr. Cedric Bryant, chief exercise physiologist for the American Council on Exercise (ACE), "An hour of physical activity appears to be necessary for optimal health. With sixty minutes of exercise a day, you can maintain health and reduce the risk of heart disease and cancer. Consumers need to hear this message as often and as consistently as possible in light of the epidemic of obesity among adults and children."[6] Ideally, the exercise should be continuous, but it could be split up into two thirty-minute sections.

Exercise is the ultimate drug. It really helps to view exercise as a drug. This perspective provides a context for just how powerful exercise truly is in the treatment of serious disease. It can also help you to recognize that, like many drugs, the dose needs to be titrated very carefully. If you are overweight, have high blood pressure, high cholesterol or diabetes then you will want to consider a daily exercise program, working up to ninety minutes per day until you normalize the problem. Of course, you should consult your doctor before starting an exercise program.

Start with walking if you are overweight. Most heavy people start with walking, and that is an excellent choice, as it is low risk and inexpensive. The major problem with walking, however, is that many people become fit relatively rapidly, but don't increase the intensity of the workouts as they become more fit. Once you become comfortable with a routine, it is important to increase the intensity in order to continue getting the benefits.

THE GREAT BIRD FLU HOAX

Increase your intensity regularly. Ideally you should exercise at an intensity that makes it somewhat difficult to talk to the person next to you. This prevents you from having to measure your pulse or use a heart-rate monitor. If you can comfortably talk to the person next to you, you aren't working hard enough to produce the benefits you need to lose weight. However, if you are using so much oxygen with your exercise that there is not enough left over to allow you to carry on a conversation at all, then you are exercising too hard and need to cut back a bit.

Consider a weight-bearing exercise. It has been my experience that non-weight-bearing exercises like bicycling are not as efficient or effective. You will typically need to exercise four times as long in these activities to receive the same benefit you would from running or using an elliptical machine.

Stick with it! The fact that we need to exercise is not news to anyone. For those who don't exercise, it's not a matter of understanding its benefits, but far more so, finding the motivation to start—and stay—on a program.

Without Proper Rest You are Bound to Get Sick

Another important key to warding off disease is making sure you get enough sleep. Just as it becomes harder for you to get your daily tasks done if you're tired, it will be harder for your body to fight the flu if it is overly fatigued. Regular rest will keep you strong and ensure that your body has the strength to fight off any potential invaders.

If you are having sleep problems, such as not being able to fall asleep, waking up too often, or not feeling well-rested when you wake up in the morning, or if you simply want to improve the quality and quantity of your sleep, try as many of the following techniques below as possible:

Avoid before-bed snacks, particularly grains and sugars. They will raise blood sugar and inhibit sleep. Later, when your blood sugar drops too low (hypoglycemia), you might wake up and not be able to fall back asleep.

Don't drink any fluids within two hours of going to bed. This will reduce the likelihood of needing to get up and go to the bathroom, or at least minimize the frequency.

But do eat a high-protein snack several hours before bed. This can provide the L-tryptophan needed to produce melatonin and serotonin. Eat a small piece of fruit at the same time—this can help the tryptophan cross the blood-brain barrier.

Avoid caffeine. A recent study showed that in some people, caffeine is not metabolized efficiently, and therefore they can feel the effects long after consuming it.[7] So an afternoon cup of coffee (or even tea) will keep some people from falling asleep. Some medications, particularly diet pills, contain caffeine.

Avoid alcohol. Although alcohol will make you drowsy, the effect is short lived and many people will often wake up several hours later, unable to fall back asleep. Alcohol will also keep you from falling into the deeper stages of sleep, where the body does most of its healing.

Avoid foods that you may be sensitive to. This is particularly true for dairy and wheat products, as they may have an effect on sleep, such as causing apnea, excess congestion, gastrointestinal upset, and gas, among others.

Lose weight. Being overweight can increase the risk of sleep apnea, which will prevent a restful night's sleep.

Make certain you are exercising regularly. Exercising for at least thirty minutes every day can help you fall asleep. However, don't exercise too close to bedtime, or it may keep you awake. Studies show that exercising in the morning is the best if you can do it.[8]

Sleep in complete darkness or as close as possible. If there is even the tiniest bit of light in the room, it can disrupt your circadian rhythm and your pineal gland's production of melatonin and serotonin. There also should be as little light in the bathroom as possible if you get up in the middle of the night. Whatever you do, keep the light off when you go to the bathroom at night. As soon as you turn on that light you will, for that night, immediately cease all production of the important sleep aid melatonin.

Get to bed as early as possible. Your adrenals, do a majority of their recharging or recovering between the hours of 11 PM and 1 AM. In addition, your gallbladder dumps toxins during this same period. If you are awake, the toxins back up into the liver, which then secondarily backs up into your entire system and causes further disruption of your health. Remember that prior to the widespread use of electricity, people would go to bed shortly after sundown, and we are still designed to do so.

Don't change your bedtime. You should go to bed, and wake up, at the same times each day, even on the weekends. This will help your body to get into a sleep rhythm and make it easier to fall asleep and get up in the morning.

Keep your bed for sleeping. If you are used to watching TV or doing work in bed, you may find it harder to relax and to think of the bed as a place to sleep.

Melatonin and its precursors. If behavioral changes do not work, it may be possible to improve your sleep by supplementing with the hormone melatonin. However, I would exercise extreme caution in using it, and only use it as a last resort, as it is a powerful hormone. Ideally, it is best to increase your melatonin levels naturally, by exposing yourself to bright sunlight in the daytime (along with full spectrum fluorescent bulbs in the winter), and sleeping in complete darkness at night. You can also use one of melatonin's precursors, L-tryptophan or 5-hydroxytryptophan (5-HTP). L-tryptophan is the safest and my preference, but it can only be obtained by prescription. However, don't be afraid or intimidated by its prescription status. It is just a simple amino acid.

Powerful Tools to Help You
Beat Stress Once and For All

We all face some stress everyday, but if stress becomes overwhelming then your body will be less able to fight off the flu and other illness. According to the Centers for Disease Control and Prevention, up to 90 percent of doctor visits may be triggered by a stress-related illness.[9, 10] Stress can lead to obesity, ulcers, heart disease and many other conditions.

Although it is still often overlooked, emotional health is absolutely essential to your physical health and healing. No matter how devoted you are to the proper diet and lifestyle, you will not achieve your body's ideal healing and preventative powers if emotional barriers stand in your way. If you are interested in learning about powerful emotional healing techniques, I reference emotional healing strategies on my website, www.mercola.com.

Sunlight—the "Miracle Drug" for Your Immune System

For several years now, the mainstream media has been helping to spread the message that the sun is bad for you. Those who believe this message, even though it contradicts every semblance of common sense, either avoid the sun as much as possible or buy lots of sunscreen to protect themselves—if you are already catching on to the "fear and consumption" campaign behind the bird flu, you will no doubt note the parallels in the "avoid the sun" fear campaign. The more fear they can instill in you about the sun, the more sunscreen you will probably buy, just as bird flu fear has led many to stock up on drugs such as Tamiflu.

It is, of course, important to use sound judgment when you

expose yourself to the sun. The level of sun exposure that goes beyond healthy and enters into the danger range is highly variable, and depends on conditions like the time of year, the paleness or darkness of your skin, the time of day, the cloud cover, and a number of other factors.

Ultimately, the goal is to receive enough sun exposure to have your skin turn the slightest bit more pink. For some, this may be as little as a few minutes; others may be able to tolerate hours in the sun without any problems. So the key for discerning optimal time in the sun is quite simple—Listen to Your Body. If you develop any excessive warmth on your skin or notice any redness, it is time to seek shade and avoid any further sun for that day.

In addition to boosting your immune system,[11, 12] sunshine makes most people feel better. Haven't you noticed how much better you feel after you've enjoyed a day at the beach or lounging in your backyard? Likewise, do you notice yourself becoming moody or depressed after it has been mostly cloudy for a few weeks or longer? Well, there's a reason for that.

The sun is one of the best ways to get a vitamin that most people are currently deficient in, vitamin D. You can get your vitamin D from three sources: food, supplements, and sunlight. Some of the best food sources of vitamin D are liver, egg yolks, cod liver oil, animal fats, and fish. But the best way to obtain vitamin D is through proper sun exposure, as vitamin D is produced by your skin in response to exposure to ultraviolet radiation from the sun.

One of the primary reasons that this is the best method is that it is virtually impossible to overdose on vitamin D from the sun, and if levels do become elevated, they lower rapidly in a matter of weeks. This is in stark contrast to the vitamin D toxicity it is possible to get from foods or supplements. It is far easier to overdose on oral vitamin D, and once your levels become elevated from oral intake, they can take months or years to normalize.

Vitamin D is most commonly known for its ability to help your body absorb calcium from the food you eat, so that you can build strong bones. However, research now reveals that its healing properties reach far beyond that. The benefits of vitamin D were mostly ignored by the scientific community until very recently, when a barrage of research started supporting the widespread utility of this important nutrient.

Vitamin D preserves muscle strength and offers some protection against diseases including:

- Heart disease[13]

- Multiple sclerosis (MS)[14]

- Diabetes[15]

- Inflammatory bowel disease[16]

- Rheumatoid arthritis[17]

- Depression[18]

- Schizophrenia[19]

- Cancer[20, 21, 22]

Evidence continues to mount that vitamin D is a very important risk reduction factor for a variety of diseases associated with internal organs, infant brain development, autoimmune diseases, and even tuberculosis.[23]

In the past, researchers estimated that the daily intake of vitamin D should be around 1,000 IU. However, most recent research on vitamin D suggests that, for acute infections, many of its health-promoting actions may require far higher doses.

According to Dr. John Cannell, high doses of vitamin D taken at the first sign of influenza can effectively reduce the severity of symptoms. He says if he had a serious infection, ". . . I wouldn't hesitate taking 200,000 units of vitamin D a day for three days."[24] Research conducted at UCLA suggests that vitamin D may also act as a potent antibiotic by increasing the body's production of naturally occurring antimicrobial peptides.[25]

> **According to Dr. John Cannell, high doses of vitamin D taken at the first sign of influenza can effectively reduce the severity of symptoms.**

Cannell asserts that "we know that vitamin D has profound effects on human immunity."[26] He suggests that more research should be conducted to see if 100,000, 200,000, or 300,000 units of vitamin D per day for several days induces antimicrobial peptides to help fight other life-threatening infections. Doses up to 600,000 units as a single dose are routinely used in Europe as "*Stoss*" therapy to prevent vitamin D deficiency, and have repeatedly been shown to be safe for short-term administration.[27]

While these doses are reasonable to consider for an acute infection in someone who is documented to be vitamin D deficient, it would be unwise to use these high oral doses as a regular program, due to the risk of oral vitamin D overdose.

However, in his newsletter, Dr. Cannell also describes another amazing method that has been used to treat infectious disease. In the 1920s, Seattle scientist Emmett Knott knew that sunlight and UV light could be used to successfully treat infectious diseases.[28, 29] The 1903 Nobel Prize in Medicine was awarded to Dr. Niels Finsen for his discovery that artificial UV radiation cured tuberculosis. Dr. Knott wondered if blood infections might be cured by irradiating the blood. He built an apparatus that removed about 5 percent of the blood volume, exposed it to UVB and UVC radiation, and then pumped the irradiated blood back into the body.

According to a book by Dr. William Campbell Douglass, *Into the Light: Tomorrow's Medicine Today,* the procedure rapidly cured both rickets and tetany. One theory is that the procedure delivers pharmacological amounts of vitamin D into the circulation (a common cause of rickets and tetany is vitamin D deficiency).[30] Many substances develop vitamin D activity when irradiated, including olive oil, cereal products, orange juice, and egg yolk. Milk used to be irradiated to fortify it with vitamin D—now the vitamin D is just added.

Hundreds of studies have been published describing the antibiotic-like actions of blood irradiation.[31] The effects of blood irradiation may be a powerful testament to the healing powers of vitamin D.

Although by now it should be obvious to you that your risk of acquiring the bird flu is highly remote, if bird flu were really a legitimate concern, or if there were any other deadly infectious threat, blood irradiation appears to be a highly effective alternative to potentially dangerous and ineffective drugs, especially when the infection is a virus for which no good drugs exist anyway.

However, by paying careful attention to sun exposure, and using UV lamps in the winter months, it is possible to maintain healthy vitamin D levels that will serve as a highly effective boost to your immune system, making it very difficult for any illness to affect you, including bird flu.

How to Make Certain You Are Getting Enough Vitamin D

Depending upon where you live, a few minutes of sun exposure on a summer day can potentially generate huge quantities of vitamin D in your body. However, just because it is sunny and hot outside, that is not necessarily an indication that you will derive benefits from the healthy UVB levels of the sun. Unfortunately, the amount of sun reaching most of the United States is only sufficient to generate a vitamin D response for about three months of the year. If your latitude is above 30 degrees north or below 30 degrees south, you will likely need vitamin D supplementation from other sources between September and mid-April.

During these months, a large share of the U.S. population doesn't come close to achieving even the absolute minimum 200 to 600 IU of vitamin D daily recommended by the National Academies' Food and Nutrition Board. A reference study done at Massachusetts General Hospital found vitamin D deficiency in over 50 percent of the subjects tested.[32] Vitamin D deficiency can manifest itself as osteomalacia (weakened muscles and bones) or rickets (characterized by malformed legs). Historically, the treatment for these conditions was cod liver oil, a rich source of vitamin D.

If you know that you're not getting enough sunlight and you're not eating enough of the foods that contain vitamin D, you may need to take vitamin D supplements. Your best choice for obtaining vitamin D would be to get regular sun exposure, as without any doubt that is the safest and most effective method. However, since for many this is simply not a practical option in the winter, my new recommendation is to consider a high-quality sunlamp that is designed to generate vitamin D levels. Sperti.com carries an excellent selection of these lamps. High-quality cod liver oil is a reasonable consideration, but if you choose this option it is essential to have your vitamin D levels checked by a qualified health care practitioner before taking any vitamin D supplementation, to confirm that you are not at risk of having an overdose.

Traditional Foods Can Have a Powerful Influence on Your Immune System

Wholesome, nutritious foods offer many benefits to your immune system and general health. However, the foods that the media has told you are healthy are, unsurprisingly, not always the foods that genuinely are healthy.

In the 1920s, Dr. Weston A. Price traveled the world in search of the fundamental characteristics of a healthy diet. He noticed that the people who relied on nutrient-dense, organic, traditional whole foods were substantially healthier than those in cultures that had started to integrate processed foods into their diet.

Dr. Price compiled his findings in his book *Nutrition and Physical Degeneration*,[33] a book that is now considered by many to be a nutritional bible. He emphasized the importance of eating foods such as butter, eggs, meat, raw milk, organ meats, and fermented foods.

Sadly, in the modern era of processed foods, many of these traditional foods have been removed from our diets, and in some cases are even accused of causing disease. For example, due to a massive disinformation campaign, many consumers believe that butter is unhealthy. Even when you visit a grocery store, butter can be difficult to locate (you may have to look down at ankle level to find it). Synthetic margarines and spreads have begun to replace a natural food that has sustained humanity for generations.

Many traditional foods have been replaced by unhealthy processed versions that are devoid of the essential micronutrients necessary to achieve high-level health. The processed food industry has been largely responsible for providing the convenience foods that have essentially forced whole foods off of most of our menus. Whatever your ancestral origin, your roots come from a traditional diet that includes high concentrations of these nutritious foods.

Historically, these foods were vital to our survival. It was less than three generations ago that animals grazed on pastures, dairy products were raw, and fermented foods were a staple in the diets of most cultures. ALL our food was grown organically, and it nearly always came from local sources. People weren't afraid of eating eggs, butter, or raw milk because they didn't have phobias about choles-terol, saturated fats, or milk contamination.

Your ancestors were healthy and robust people. They may have had to contend with harsh winters, contaminated water, and starva-tion, but they didn't experience the epidemic of diet-caused chronic degenerative diseases that we face today. In today's Western cultures, we don't face the same hardships that our ancestors did, but many of our contemporary challenges come from the poor quality food many of us choose to eat. If you really want to keep from falling ill with bird flu, or for that matter any other kind of illness, then switching to a healthier diet may be the most important change you can make.

> **If you really want to keep from falling ill with bird flu, or for that matter any other kind of illness, then switching to a healthier diet may be the most important change you can make.**

Raw Milk and Pasteurized Milk— The Story You Haven't Been Told

The evolution of the contemporary diet of highly processed food is a single story repeated over and over; natural, healthy, whole foods are stripped of their essential nutrients and made unhealthy, and then an inferior synthetic supplement is added to partially compen-sate for the damage that processing does.

The story of pasteurized milk is probably the prime example of the kind of slapped-on Band-Aid "solution" that conventional food processors use to validate their approach.

Ron Schmid, ND, author of the book *The Untold Story of Milk*,[34] describes how a century ago, milk began to become contaminated because of the way the cows were fed and treated. That was the beginning of the era when cows were forced to remain indoors and fed diets high in grain. Normally, cows graze on plush grass, and they also benefit by absorbing the vitamin D from the sun while they do so.

When cows are raised consistently with the requirements of their genetic heritage, they produce very safe, healing, and nourishing milk. But cows that are kept in confinement and fed grains that they were never designed to eat tend to be prone to acquiring infections contaminate their milk. The pasteurization process was introduced as a Band-Aid attempt to solve the dairy industry's problem without going to the expense and inconvenience of putting cows back on pasture.

Gradually, as more cows were condemned to a life sentence in a factory farm jail, raw milk progressively lost out to commercial, pasteurized milk. As a result, nearly everyone in the United States has been forced into buying this damaged substitute, rather than whole, raw milk.

Raw milk is an outstanding source of nutrients, including beneficial bacteria such as *Lactobacillus Acidophilus*, vitamins, and enzymes, and it is one of the best available sources of calcium.

While pasteurization certainly can destroy potentially harmful and infectious bacteria, it also destroys the milk's beneficial bacteria, along with many of its nutritious components. The pasteurization process also significantly alters the structure of the milk proteins into a far less healthy version, by distorting the structure of the protein.

Pasteurizing milk not only destroys the functional activity of its enzymes, but it also diminishes levels of vitamins such as B12 and B6. In addition, it kills the healthy bacteria normally found in the milk. Raw milk left out will sour naturally and ferment into cheeses, but pasteurized milk will rot. This is because the beneficial bacteria in the raw milk helps to keep pathogens (including "bad" bacteria like listeria) under control. In other word, raw milk is loaded with its own "immunity," which prevents pathogens from proliferating.

Then, of course, there is the issue of the antibiotics, pesticides, and growth hormones and the fact that nearly all commercial dairy cows are raised on grains, not the grass they were designed to eat. If cows are outside grazing on grass, not only are the cows healthier, so is the milk. In fact the composition of the fats in the milk also improves, especially the amount of conjugated linoleic acid (CLA), which may help reduce the risk of cancer.

The Many Health Benefits of Raw Milk

Pasteurized cow's milk is the number one allergenic food in this country. It has been associated with a number of symptoms and illnesses including:

- Diarrhea
- Cramps
- Bloating
- Gas
- Gastrointestinal bleeding
- Iron-deficiency anemia
- Skin rashes
- Allergies
- Colic in infants
- Osteoporosis
- Increased tooth decay
- Growth problems in children
- Heart disease
- Cancer
- Atherosclerosis
- Acne
- Recurrent ear infections in children
- Type 1 diabetes
- Rheumatoid arthritis
- Infertility
- Leukemia
- Arthritis
- Autism

Raw milk, on the other hand, is not associated with any of these problems, and even people who have been allergic to pasteurized milk for many years can typically tolerate and even thrive on raw milk.

For most people, raw milk from grass-fed cows is truly one of the most profoundly healthy foods you can consume, and you'll feel the difference once you start to drink it. I have treated many patients from Eastern Europe, and nearly all of them recall how they were raised on raw milk from pastured cows that provided superior taste and health benefits. They are generally shocked to learn that this nourishing food is not readily available in the United States.

In nearly all states but California, it is illegal to sell raw milk commercially. However, in many states throughout the United States, there are legal workarounds called cow share programs that allow individuals to purchase a share in the cow and pay the farmer for milking their cow. Cow share programs have survived multiple legal assaults, and can provide a practical alternative for many to secure this important form of nutrition. For more information about finding raw milk, you can take a look at www.realmilk.com.

Sugar and Scurvy—A Classic Example of the Power of Whole Foods

In his book *Sugar Blues*,[35] Bill Dufty points out numerous examples of physical diseases and psychological disorders that can be traced back to diets that are deficient in whole unprocessed foods, and dominated by highly processed fats and sugars. He notes that "men who lived away from the land in new cities or on board ships discovering new worlds ate food that was increasingly refined; eventually they sickened."[36]

One glaring example he notes is that "by 1662, sugar consumption in England had zoomed from zero to some 16 million pounds a year, this in little over two centuries. Then, in 1665, London was swept by a plague."[37] You may recall from chapter 1 that many now believe that two of the major factors leading to the spread of this great plague were poor hygiene and immune systems that were weakened as a result of improper diet.

Shortly after the plague, Dr. Thomas Willis noticed a connection between scurvy and sugar, over a hundred years before the discovery of vitamin C by Scottish naval surgeon James Lind in 1747. "I do much disapprove things preserved or very much seasoned with sugar," Willis wrote. "I judge the invention of it and its immoderate use to have very much contributed to the vast increase in scurvy in this last age . . ."[38] In the seventeenth and eighteenth centuries, as natural sugars such as fruits or honey were being replaced more and more by refined sugar, the British dominated and controlled the sugar trade while thousands of their sailors were dying of scurvy.

Even after Lind discovered the connection between citrus and scurvy, it took almost fifty years before the Royal Navy introduced lemons to the sailors' rations. According to Dufty, in between the time Lind made his discovery and the time lemons were added to the sailors' rations in 1795, an additional 100,000 sailors died from scurvy.[39]

Nearly a century and half later, in the summer of 1933, a wise group of native Americans taught Dr. Weston A. Price that the adrenal glands of the moose can be used as a remedy for scurvy. They knew that food was their medicine, and turned to natural solutions such as nutrient dense foods like organ meats and herbs as powerful remedies.

The Vikings, the Phoenicians, and the sailors of the Far East never experienced outbreaks of scurvy during their sea travels. They were able to ward off scurvy because their diets included foods such as beans, lentils, sprouted seeds, salted cabbage, or pickled vegetables in brine.[40] Captain Cook took sixty barrels of sauerkraut onto his ship for his second trip around the world. Not one case of scurvy was reported on this long voyage.[41]

The workers building the Great Wall of China supplemented their rice-based diets with salted cabbage. Julius Caesar's soldiers ate whole grains supplemented with cabbage or other vegetables. At that time, cabbage was known for its preventative and healing properties.[42] In the thirteenth century, Hungarians transformed cabbage into sauerkraut, which became one of the staple foods of Germany and Eastern Europe.

Another testimony to the power of whole foods on scourges and epidemics is that during the American Civil War, Dr. John Hay Terrill was able to reduce the death rate from small pox from 90 percent to 5 percent by giving his patients sauerkraut.[43]

Korean Sauerkraut May Be a Powerful Key to the Treatment and Prevention of Bird Flu

For generations, Koreans have believed that kimchi, a pungent fermented cabbage that is traditional to their culture, has properties that ward off disease. In order to prove its health benefits, kimchi is now being studied extensively by scientists in South Korea.[44] Scientists at Seoul National University in South Korea fed an extract of this spicy variation of sauerkraut to thirteen chickens infected with the highly pathogenic bird flu virus (H5N1).[45] Studies have found that the virus can infect the gut as well as the respiratory tract,[46] and the researchers hoped that certain compounds in kimchi would help the birds recover. It seems as though they were right—eleven of the chickens recovered from the disease.

Professor Sa-ouk Kang, one of the researchers who conducted the study, said, "We don't know exactly whether the kimchi lactobacillus itself is killing the virus or strengthening cells . . . What is certain at this point is that when we feed kimchi lactobacillus to bird-flu infected chickens, they are cured."[47]

Following this experiment, the results were repeated in a larger study on at least 200,000 Korean chickens.[48] The birds were fed a specific compound found in the kimchi (a culture filtrate of the bacteria Leuconostoc Kimchii).

Given the overall benefits of the biologically active compounds in kimchi, it should be no surprise to discover that this traditional food could have powerful healing attributes. Research indicates that the combination of the many ingredients in kimchi could offer health benefits such as:

- Antibiotic properties

- Anticarcinogenic properties

- Boosting the immune system

- Antioxidants

- Balancing gut bacteria[49]

Based upon the findings of the South Korean study, even *Men's Health Magazine* recommended constructing a pandemic kit including "... a few cans of the [Korean] sauerkraut; it's packed with lactic-acid bacteria, shown by Korean researchers to speed recovery of chickens infected with avian flu."[50]

Sauerkraut and kimchi sales have increased dramatically following the study.[51] According to Chris Smith, vice president of marketing for Frank's Sauerkraut, "If you look at a 19th century Old Farmer's Almanac you'll find recipes for sauerkraut to treat virtually every ailment under the sun. Now in the 21st century it's been cited as having cancer fighting abilities and may be a cure for avian flu. It's truly one of the most unassuming super foods ever created. We expect to see sales go through the roof this Fall."[52]

Fermented Foods Offer Many Surprises

Before canning machines, refrigerators, and freezers had been invented, our ancestors needed some form of food preservation to get them through times when they did not have access to fresh foods. But even though fermentation was initially used as a way to preserve foods, our ancestors also learned that fermented foods also had powerful healing properties.[53] If you thought that the only benefit of fermentation is to preserve foods, you will be surprised by the many health benefits they offer.

Sandor Ellix Katz, author of *Wild Fermentation*, says that "fermented foods and drinks are quite literally alive with flavor and nutrition."[54] According to Katz, "The process of fermentation makes food more digestible and nutritious. Live, unpasteurized, fermented foods also carry beneficial bacteria directly into our digestive systems, where they exist symbiotically, breaking down food and aiding digestion."[55]

The Food and Agriculture Organization (FAO) have published a document series about the many important values of fermented foods.[56] They found that:

- The lowering of the pH inhibits the growth of food spoiling or poisoning bacteria and destroys certain pathogens[57]

- Certain lactic acid bacteria (e.g. *Lactobacillus acidophilus*) that grow during the fermentation process have been found to produce antibiotics and bacteriocins[58, 59, 60, 61, 62]

- The beneficial health effects of lactic acid bacteria on the intestinal flora are well documented[63, 64]

- Substances in fermented foods have been found to have a protective effect against the development of cancer[65]

Research has shown that, in some foods, fermentation increases certain vitamins such as thiamine, niacin, riboflavin, nicotinic acid, folic acid, and biotin and raises the protein content or improves the balance of essential amino acids or their availability.[66,67] Fermentation is a traditional method of reducing the microbial contamination of porridges in Kenya.[68] A study in Tanzania showed that, due to the inhibition of pathogenic bacteria by lactic acid forming bacteria, children fed with fermented gruels had a 33 percent lower incidence of diarrhea than those fed unfermented gruels.[69]

Different fermentation processes create a variety of foods and drinks. Because of the practical nature of using lactic acid fermentation, I will highlight some of the many benefits of this specific method. You may already be familiar with some fairly traditional foods that are produced through lacto-fermentation, such as sauerkraut, yogurt, kefir, sour cream, sourdough bread, miso, natto, and tempeh.

The beneficial bacteria that grow during this fermentation process produce lactic acid, which creates an environment that discourages the growth of undesirable microorganisms. This process serves as an excellent natural preservative, preventing spoilage. But it also results in powerful health benefits.

Getting Healthy with Lacto-Fermented Foods

Lacto-fermented vegetables, such as sauerkraut, are known for their medicinal qualities, including their ability to relieve intestinal problems and constipation. Keeping your gut healthy is one of the powerful keys to maintaining good health. Lacto-fermented foods help support your digestive process by normalizing the acidity of your stomach. They have also been used to help treat or prevent diseases such as smallpox and scurvy.

In her book *Nourishing Traditions*, Sally Fallon says that during the nineteenth century, European doctors prescribed sauerkraut to treat a variety of different ailments, including "enlarged spleen, hemorrhoids, constipation, nervous troubles and hysteria. In Germany and Poland sauerkraut juice and juice of fermented cucumbers are still used to treat enteritis."[70]

The health-promoting microorganisms that are formed during lacto-fermentation also produce beneficial enzymes, as well as antibiotic and anticarcinogenic substances.[71, 72]

The lactic acid formed during fermentation also helps break down proteins, thus making them easier to absorb. One study also found significantly better absorption of iron from a mix of lacto-fermented vegetables, as compared to the same mix of fresh vegetables.[73]

Lacto-fermented foods also contain large amounts of choline, a nutrient that helps lower blood pressure.[74] Sauerkraut also contains acetylcholine, which helps to promote calmness and sleep.[75, 76] In addition, acetylcholine promotes peristalsis in the intestinal tract, which helps improve elimination.[77]

Consumption of lacto-fermented vegetables has been positively associated with low rates of asthma, skin problems, and auto-immune disorders.[78] The same study found that use of raw milk and avoidance of vaccinations added to the protective effects.[79]

Finnish researchers found that fermented cabbage is healthier for you than raw or cooked cabbage.[80] Fermenting cabbage produces powerful compounds called isothiocyanates, which may help prevent the growth of cancer.[81] Cruciferous vegetables such as cabbage and broccoli contain glucosinolate, which breaks down to isothiocyanates during the fermentation process. Other studies have demonstrated that isothiocyanates encourage precancerous cells in the digestive system to self-destruct (a process called apoptosis). A team of Polish and U.S. researchers also found that glucosinolates may help reduce the risk of breast cancer in women.[82]

As has been noted, kimchi is made through the process of lacto-fermentation, and the lactic acid created during its fermentation appears to help chickens fight the highly pathogenic bird flu virus.

Lacto-fermentation can reduce the amount of certain (naturally-occurring) antinutritional components of certain foods such as grains, soy, and some vegetables. One study found an 87 percent reduction of nitrates in cabbage and a 70 percent reduction of oxalic acid in beets after fermentation.[83] It is important to ferment soy in order to break down the thyroid blocking goitrogens. Asian cultures have learned the importance of fermenting soy, and have developed a variety of traditional fermented soy foods in their diet (such as miso, tempeh, and tamari).

Unfortunately, many commercial soy foods are not fermented, which means that they are not only difficult to digest but actively harmful to your health.[84] The focus on soy that has been pervasive in the health food industry throughout North America has fooled even conscientious individuals, and many professionals, into believing they are purchasing a healthy product when they are not.

Even though I caution people about eating grains, traditionally prepared sourdough breads, which are fermented with lactic acid bacteria and yeasts, are a much healthier choice than commercial bread because they are much easier to digest. Lactic acid fermentation breaks down foods, making them more easily digestible.[85, 86] Also, because the carbohydrates in lactic-fermented foods are broken down, they do not make heavy demands on the pancreas. Studies have shown that the glycemic response to baked goods made with sourdough is significantly lowered.[87, 88] Even when grains are properly prepared, though, be sure to eat them in moderation.

Traditionally, grains were always fermented before consumption: recipes for sourdough breads, pancakes, and biscuits included fermentation. Throughout Europe, grains were soaked overnight, sometimes for as long as several days, in water or sour milk before they were cooked and served as porridge or gruel. Grains carefully prepared in this manner deliver far more nutritional value and are, of course, much easier to digest than denatured processed foods.

Soaking grains also helps break down phytic acid, which can block the absorption of certain minerals such as zinc, calcium, iron, and magnesium. When preparing your oatmeal from large rolled organic oats for breakfast, it is best to soak the oats overnight in water so that the oats can be more easily digested.[89]

Integrating fermented foods into your diet may not be as much work as it seems, as many fermented foods can be purchased and require no preparation. However, it is less expensive and typically healthier if you prepare these foods yourself, so that you ensure they are as fresh and healthy as possible. It is important to note that if you want to fully benefit from eating fermented foods, you should ensure that they are unpasteurized, as pasteurization can destroy the important micronutrients that provide the benefits of fermented foods.

Yogurt—What You Don't Know May Hurt You

Some individuals prefer to consume fermented raw milk in the form of yogurt or kefir. Because yogurt and kefir are fermented, they can be much easier to digest.

Lactic acid bacteria is also formed in dairy products during the fermentation process. Lactic acid bacteria found in fermented dairy products may release compounds that help prevent infections and tumors.[90, 91, 92] Fermentation can also increase certain vitamins in dairy products (especially B vitamins such as folic acid, riboflavin, niacin, thiamin, and biotin).[93, 94] Feeding mice with milk fermented by lactic acid bacteria led to significant increases in various immune responses.[95]

Fermented dairy products, such as kefir and yogurt, are well known for their ability to provide beneficial flora (probiotics) to the intestinal tract and aid in digestion. Probiotics have been shown to provide many health benefits, including increasing resistance to intestinal infections, stimulating the immune system, and possibly protecting against cancer.[96] Researchers believe that the intestinal lining of your gut comprises approximately 70 percent of your immune system, which is one of the reasons it's so important to encourage the growth of friendly microflora with fermented foods. In addition, the fermentation process in dairy products also helps increase levels of the anticarcinogenic conjugated linoleic acid (CLA).[97]

Many cultures around the world use their own traditional fermented dairy products to treat disease. In Russia, the fermented milk product koumiss has been used to treat tuberculosis.[98] In India, dahi, another traditional fermented dairy product, is used to treat dyspepsia, dysentery, and various intestinal disorders.[99] Consumption of fermented dairy products may provide protection against diseases organisms[100] and could also help protect against the incidence of colon cancer.[101]

Yogurt is produced by the bacterial fermentation of milk. It is the fermentation of milk sugar (lactose) into lactic acid that gives yogurt its texture and taste. Yogurt is an excellent source of calcium, phosphorous, riboflavin (vitamin B2), iodine, vitamin B12, pantothenic acid (vitamin B5), zinc, potassium, protein, and molybdenum.[102] Yogurt is also very helpful in the treatment and prevention of antibiotic associated diarrhea,[103] and has a beneficial effect on the common problem of persistent diarrhea in children,[104] as the healthy bacteria in the yogurt help to normalize the gut ecology.

Japanese researchers conducted a study to see if yogurt containing two friendly strains of bacteria, *Lactobacillus bulgaricus* and *Streptococcus thermophilus*, would help reduce levels of hydrogen sulfide, a major cause of bad breath. Bad breath is frequently a sign that there is a problem in the digestive system. Researchers found that hydrogen sulfide levels decreased in 80 percent of the participants who ate three ounces of yogurt twice daily for six weeks.[105, 106] They also noticed decreased levels of plaque and the gum disease gingivitis.

The use of healthy bacteria, like those found in yogurt, to treat illnesses like bird flu is also supported by a study published in the *Journal of Nutrition*. Researchers found that lactobacillus casei, a strain of friendly bacteria that can be found in yogurt significantly improved immune response and the ability to fight off pneumonia.[107] Research has also shown that increased yogurt consumption may enhance immune response and increase resistance to immune-related diseases.[108]

Many people don't realize, however, that commercial yogurts don't necessarily provide all of these benefits. Most commercial yogurts don't have any active friendly bacteria in them, because most companies pasteurize the product, killing the microorganisms.[109] Rather than buying yogurt at a grocery store, consider purchasing your yogurt from a health food store and reading the label to make sure it is a brand that has live active cultures or, better yet, make it yourself, which is relatively easy to do. A recipe for yogurt, along with recipes for several of the other foods mentioned in this chapter, can be found in the appendix.

Kefir—Growing in Popularity

Another fermented dairy product that is gaining popularity in North America is called kefir. If you're unfamiliar with kefir, the easiest way to describe it is to say that it is very much like yogurt, but not quite as thick, so you can drink it like a liquid. Like yogurt, kefir can be purchased at your grocery or health food store, but most commercial brands are loaded with sugars that virtually destroy its value as a health food. Fortunately, kefir is also very easy to make, so you can avoid these problems by making it yourself.

Kefir comes from the Central Asian Caucasus Mountains. In Turkish, the word *kefir* means "good feeling," which is not surprising considering the fact that kefir is loaded with health-promoting enzymes and friendly microorganisms. Kefir has a tart flavor that many would describe as refreshing, and it differs from yogurt in that it contains beneficial yeast as well as the friendly bacteria.

Kefir and yogurt contain different types of bacteria as well. Yogurt contains bacteria that help keep your digestive system clean, and provides nourishment for the friendly bacteria that already are present. Kefir actually colonizes your intestinal tract with friendly microorganisms that combine to build and strengthen your immune system, which helps to increase your resistance to intestinal infections. In addition, several studies have investigated the antitumor activity of kefir.[110, 111, 112]

Kefir is also rich in nutrients such as vitamins K, B1, B6 (pyridoxine), B9 (folic acid), B12, and B7 (biotin).[113] Biotin helps your body absorb other B vitamins,[114] and maintaining adequate levels of B vitamins in your body increases energy and helps support your kidneys, liver, nervous system, and skin. Kefir contains phosphorus as well, an important mineral that helps with the utilization of carbohydrates, fats, and proteins for cell growth, maintenance and energy.[115]

Recipes for sauerkraut, yogurt, and kefir can be found in the appendix. When fermenting dairy products, be sure to use raw milk. Also, depending upon what you are fermenting, be sure to avoid chlorinated water and iodized salt, as they can interfere with the fermentation process (this applies to sauerkraut, for example).

Fresh, Wholesome, Natural Ingredients

All of the foods and lifestyle changes that have been discussed in this book can help boost your immune system to the extent that you will minimize your concerns concerns about catching the bird flu or any other serious infectious. As a bonus, you will also be free of the chronic, degenerative diseases that are the real epidemics of modern society—if you bear one important factor in mind:

> **The foods you eat, and the ingredients you use, need to be fresh, local, and free of pesticides. Food that passes through the conventional system of factory farms is more prone to being diseased, has had most of its nutrients destroyed, has been treated with dangerous chemicals, and has traveled too far to be fresh.**

If the bird flu scare has any benefit, it may be that it will cause people to look more closely at the system that produces their food, and move away from the "bird jails" and factory farming systems that are the true root of the problem.

7

A SILVER LINING

Could the Bird Flu Be a Blessing in Disguise?

"The true costs of quick food must include the costs of poor health, lost dignity in work, degraded landscapes, and ethical and moral decay in business matters, including international trade and investment. We are paying a tremendously high price for the time saved by choosing quick food."[1]

—JOHN IKERD,
Professor Emeritus, University of Missouri

The bird flu has been used as an excuse to instill even more fear in a population already feeling threatened by a host of media-manufactured threats. But it's possible that this could backfire and cause people to take a hard look at the source behind the spread of the fear. There are, in fact, genuine concerns regarding the progressive decrease in the quality of your food supply. If people ask the right questions, the bird flu could serve as a clarion call, rather than another reason to remain paralyzed with fear.

> There are, in fact, genuine concerns regarding the progressive decrease in the quality of your food supply. If people ask the right questions, the bird flu could serve as a clarion call, rather than another reason to remain paralyzed with fear.

After having examined the risks in factory farming in chapters 3 and 4, it should be clear that the need to support a healthier agricultural system is a critical issue for assuring the future safety of your food supply. Why should you support the large multinational food corporations, when their primary focus is on increasing the profits of their shareholders, without any regard to the potential impact their practices might have on the consumers they serve? Is the convenience they offer enough of a benefit for you to support risky and unethical agricultural practices by purchasing their factory food?

Over the last few years, you have been bombarded with bad news about food contamination (such as E. coli, foot-and-mouth disease, and many others). If you've joined the ranks of people who are questioning the quality of your food, you're far from being alone. The bird flu threat may be the last straw for many who have been questioning why these conditions were ever allowed to exist in the first place. In response to this dilemma, many are choosing to purchase their food from local farms where they practice time-tested traditional methods of farming.

Why You Should Buy Organic

Highly processed and chemicalized foods that mimic whole foods do not provide the nutritional benefits that their traditional counterparts do. Not only are most contemporary foods loaded with preservatives and artificial flavorings, they are missing important vitamins, minerals, enzymes, micronutrients, and friendly bacteria that have historically contributed to good health.

The decision to purchase organic food over conventionally grown food is a personal one, and as you walk through the supermarket, many of which are now adding organic sections, you will likely ask the question: Is organic food really worth the extra money?

Organic food is certainly growing in popularity The global market for organic foods is expected to expand from $26 billion in 2001 to $80 billion in 2008.[2] Growth in sales of organic food has been 15 percent to 21 percent each year, compared with 2 percent to 4 percent for total food sales.[3]

Organic farming differs from conventional farming in the methods used to grow crops. Where traditional farmers apply chemical fertilizers to the soil to grow their crops, organic farmers build the soil with natural fertilizers. Traditional farmers use pesticides to control insects and disease, while organic farmers use natural methods such as insect predators and barriers. Traditional farmers contain weed growth by applying synthetic herbicides, but organic farmers use crop rotation, tillage, hand weeding, cover crops, and mulches.

The result is that conventionally grown food is often tainted with chemical residues, which can be harmful. There is debate over whether dietary exposure to pesticides at the levels typically found on food is dangerous, but you should use caution. The Environmental Protection Agency (EPA) considers 60 percent of herbicides, 90 percent of fungicides, and 30 percent of insecticides to be carcinogenic.[4]

Pesticides can have many negative influences on your health, including damage to your nervous system, disruption of your endocrine system, and immune system suppression. Since organic foods are not treated with pesticides, eating them allows you to limit your exposure to toxic chemicals that have been linked to cancer, leukemia, Parkinson's disease, infertility, birth defects, and adverse neurological and neurobehavioral effects.

Choosing organic food also increases your chances of eating more nutritious food. The greater the nutrient content of the food you eat, the more likely that you'll keep your immune system strong so that you can ward off any disease, even ones like bird flu.

On average, conventional produce has only 83 percent of the

nutrients of organic produce. Studies have found significantly higher levels of nutrients such as vitamin C, iron, magnesium, and phosphorus. Organic crops also contain fewer nitrates, which can be carcinogenic.[5]

Organic farming is better for the environment as well. In 2006, research published in the *Proceedings of the National Academy of Sciences* provided strong evidence to support the claim that organic agriculture is superior to conventional farming in this regard.[6] According to the authors of the study, "Conventional agriculture has made tremendous improvements in crop yield but at large costs to the environment . . . In response to environmental concerns, organic agriculture has become an increasingly popular option."[7]

New Research Proves Organic Farming is Healthier for You

The benefits of less intensive agricultural practices have been confirmed by a progressively increasing number of studies. In September 2005, The Organic Center for Education and Promotion released the results of an extensive analysis that showed that organic farming practices can decrease the risk of dangerous mycotoxin contamination in foods, especially grain-based products.[8]

Dr. Chuck Benbrook notes that conventional farmers often "apply more nitrogen fertilizer than is really needed. Fungi and bacteria often thrive in a farming environment that has excess nutrients in it . . . The opposite is true for organically based systems which rarely have an excess supply of nitrogen . . ."[9] He adds that the fungicides used in conventional farming may even make the problem worse, because they are "designed to kill certain classes of fungi . . . It will stress [other fungi], but not kill them . . . This sub-lethal dose can trigger mycotoxin formation in some of the other fungi that are not controlled."[10]

Studies have also shown that organically grown strawberries inhibit cancer cells more successfully than their conventional equivalent.[11, 12] Organic wheat and rice have little or no detectable pesticide residue,[13] and children who switch to an organic diet show an immediate reduction in pesticide exposure.[14]

While it's all well and good to have less exposure to toxic chemicals and more nutrients, there is one benefit you will immediately enjoy: organic foods taste better! Organic vegetables and fruits are sweeter and more compact because they have a higher dry matter and mineral content. Possibly as a result of this, they also show better storage quality during winter keeping.[15]

Farm animals from organically raised herds experience far fewer metabolic diseases such as lipidosis, arthritis, mastitis, and milk fever. Milk and meat from organically reared animals contains more CLA (conjugated linoleic acid), which, as you will recall, is thought to prevent cancer in humans.[16, 17, 18, 19]

Conventional Vegetables Still Better Than No Vegetables at All

There is little question that organic foods are superior to nonorganic ones. However, I see many patients who are not eating any vegetables because they either cannot afford organic produce or have found it too difficult to obtain. However, it is important to understand that it is better to eat nonorganic vegetables than no vegetables at all.

Similarly, it is also important to realize that fresh nonorganic vegetables will be better than wilted or rotten organic vegetables, which are occasionally the only ones available in smaller organic produce stands. There are many highly perishable nutrients that degrade with time and exposure to air and ultraviolet radiation. If the organic vegetables are seriously damaged, then it would be far wiser to eat fresh, undamaged non-organic vegetables.

Fortunately, as the demand for organic food increases, the prices will drop and the supply will increase, making it far easier to obtain relatively inexpensive high-quality organic produce.

If you must buy conventional produce, there are ways to reduce your pesticide exposure. Thoroughly washing all fruits and vegetables will help, although all pesticide residues cannot be removed by washing. You can also remove the outer layer of leaves or peel vegetables if possible. Another alternative is to grow your own vegetables, although this takes space and time, and is subject to climate considerations.

Another option is to buy organic produce selectively, as certain foods tend to have higher or lower amounts of pesticides. The following foods tend to have the highest levels of pesticides:

FRUITS AND VEGETABLES[20] HIGH IN PESTICIDES	
FRUIT	**VEGETABLES**
Peaches	Spinach
Apples	Bell Peppers
Strawberries	Celery
Nectarines	Potatoes
Pears	Hot Peppers
Cherries	
Red Raspberries	
Imported Grapes	

These foods tend to be lower in pesticide levels.

Fruit	Vegetables
Pineapples	Cauliflower
Plantains	Brussels Sprouts
Mangoes	Asparagus
Bananas	Radishes
Watermelon	Broccoli
Plums	Onions
Kiwi	Okra
Blueberries	Cabbage
Papaya	Eggplant
Grapefruit	
Avacado	

Look Beyond the Label—Some Practical Cautions About Choosing Organic Foods

You need to exercise some caution when buying organic food. Just because a food is certified as organic and is sold at Whole Foods does not necessarily mean that it is healthy.

Organic Sugar and Processed Foods

Any highly processed organic foods, or ones that have sugar in them, are especially suspect, even if it is organic cane sugar. It is still sugar and can disrupt your immune system, as was discussed in the previous chapter.

If you buy organic potato chips, French fries, boxed crackers, cookies, or cereal, chances are they are going to be just as bad for you as their conventional counterparts. Whether such foods are conventionally or organically grown won't change the fact that these foods can contain high amounts of chemical additives, or another very toxic chemical, acrylamide, which is formed during processing.

Acrylamide is formed in certain foods by what is known as the Maillard reaction, in which amino acids react with sugars when foods are heated to more than 120°C. According to the U.S. Environmental Protection Agency's (EPA) Web site, "The EPA . . . has classified acrylamide as a Group B2, probable human carcinogen."[21] The European Commission Scientific Committee on Food believes that ". . . levels of acrylamide should be as low as reasonably achievable."[22]

Genetically Modified Foods

One piece of information you are unlikely to see clearly marked on any label is whether or not any of the ingredients are genetically modified foods. GM foods did not exist prior to 1995, but 70 percent of processed foods now have genetically modified foods in them.[23]

According to the president of the Campaign to Label Genetically Engineered Foods, Craig Winters:

> The Grocery Manufacturers Association and the mainstream food industry have opposed labeling genetically engineered foods. Why? Because they know that if these foods are labeled that customers will start asking questions such as "Have these foods been safety tested?" The answer to that question is "no'"and therefore consumers are not going to want to be guinea pigs in this giant feeding experiment. In every nation around the world where labeling regulations have been implemented, companies have switched to non-genetically engineered sources since they know consumers will reject these risky foods.[24]

Corporations have fought long and hard to keep this information off of food labels, in an attempt not to alarm customers.[25] As a result, the FDA does not require such labeling in nearly every case. [26]

You should definitely be concerned, however. There have been no studies done with humans to show what happens when genetically modified foods are consumed. The FDA has naively and dangerously *assumed* that these modified foods are equivalent to the original foods and do not require any studies to have them approved, despite the fact that this technology has never before existed in the history of the world.[27]

Fortunately, there are a number of simple ways to identify and avoid GM foods:

- Reduce or eliminate processed foods.

- Avoid foods with ingredients that are corn or soy derivatives, such as corn flour and meal, dextrin, starch, soy sauce, margarine, and tofu (to name a few).

- Check produce stickers on fruit—GM foods will have five numbers, the first one being the number 8.

- Buy organic, as current certification does not allow any genetically modified foods to be classified as organic.

However, someday soon, even those measures may not be enough. GM crops are plants, and they mix and interbreed with other crops, as all plants do. Large numbers of organic seeds have been contaminated with GM material, to the extent that the North Dakota organic certification agency, Farm Verified Organic, posited that "the GM pollution of American commodities is now so pervasive, we believe it is not possible for farmers in North America to source seed free from it."[28]

I perceive this as one of the most serious threats to the future of food that this world has ever seen. My next book will focus entirely on this issue.

Organic Beef

Certified organic beef is not necessarily as healthy as grass-fed, non-factory farmed beef. Most of the organic beef I have seen has been fed organic corn, which still has many of the same problems that have traditionally been associated with eating beef. Most grass-fed beef uses feed crops that are not sprayed with pesticides, but the ranchers are not always able to afford the expensive organic certification process. To date, there is no regulatory system in place to fully monitor grass-fed beef, so your best bet is to buy from local farms where you can see for yourself whether or not they pasture their animals.

Organic Milk

The primary concern with milk is not whether it is organic, but whether it is raw. You can have milk from the best grass-fed cow, but if it is pasteurized, then the milk is damaged. Organic damaged milk is not necessarily, and usually isn't, the best milk to purchase. Just as with beef, most of the time if you find a local farmer providing raw milk from grass-fed cows, it will likely have all the characteristics of organic milk, but the farmers may not have been able to afford the certification process.

As with purchasing any of your food, but especially with milk, it would be wise to personally visit the farmer so you, not some government agency, can certify that the living conditions of the cows are ones that you are comfortable with, and that the farmer has a high level of integrity and commitment to healthy living practices.

Organic Grains

Naturally, you will need to be cautious about consuming too many organic grains, even whole grains. Remember that over 75 percent of the U.S. population would likely benefit from a severe reduction of their grain intake, as it is one of the primary ways insulin is elevated. You will particularly want to avoid grains if you are overweight, have high blood pressure or high cholesterol, or are diabetic or prediabetic.

Organic Chicken and Eggs

Factory farming has caused many consumers to question their chicken and egg choices at the grocery store. As a result, some companies are marketing "free run," "cage free," "omega 3," "organic," or "natural" eggs. You can also find "organic," "natural," "hormone free," and "antibiotic free" chicken.

But many of these labels can be deceiving. For example, some farmers jokingly call "free run" eggs "balcony chickens" because the chickens simply have to have access to the outdoors. Therefore, in order to meet the criteria, some chicken operations simply build a "balcony" on their barn. That's one way the corporations still get away with selling you inferior products, even if you're sensitized to the importance of this factor.

In the "organic" commercial chicken and egg industry, the chickens are usually raised indoors. They may run free in a barn, but they are not outside running around on pasture eating grass, weeds, bugs, and worms and absorbing the benefits of the sun (vitamin D).

USDA certified organic eggs may be slightly better than

conventional eggs (at least they're not given arsenic!), but the chickens probably haven't been left outside to eat naturally growing foods. The term *organic* can be used very loosely in the production of eggs, chicken, pork, meat, and dairy. Although there are exceptions, the large corporations that produce massive quantities of "organic" eggs, chicken, meat, pork, and dairy generally don't pasture their animals. Sadly, it can be a very misleading term.

The information you read in earlier chapters regarding the diseases and toxins that lace factory-farmed chicken may cause you to believe that you should give up eggs altogether. However, when eggs are purchased from local farms that pasture their poultry, rather than from confinement operations, you will avoid the potentially dangerous food produced by diseased chickens, as locally raised pastured poultry is among the healthiest of foods that you can choose to eat.

Eggs—One of Nature's Most Wholesome Foods

Since the dawn of civilization, eggs have been celebrated as a symbol of fertility, creation, and new life. There is archaeological evidence for egg consumption dating back to the Neolithic age. Eggs are unique in that they contain nearly every known nutrient essential to humans. This is not hard to understand once you realize that nature designed them as total life-support systems for developing chicks.

Even though eggs have been demonized for several decades now, new information has surfaced that helps support the fact that they are an extremely healthy food. A review published in the British Nutrition Foundation's *Nutrition Bulletin* examined more than thirty studies conducted over the past thirty years, with more than half published in the past decade. It concluded that the dietary cholesterol in eggs "has no clinically significant impact" on coronary heart disease (CHD) risk.[29] A Harvard study cited in the review, which included more than 100,000 subjects, found no significant difference in cardiovascular disease risk between groups consuming less than one egg per day and those consuming more than one egg per day.[30]

According to Donald J. McNamara, PhD, "The decades' worth of studies examined in this review underscore the many positive effects eggs have on our health. Based on the current evidence, healthy adults should feel confident that they can enjoy eggs daily without fear of cholesterol or heart disease."[31]

Egg whites contain a very high-quality protein, as they have exactly the right combination of essential amino acids required to build healthy animal tissues. The protein in an egg is so ideal that it is used as the standard against which other protein foods are judged. The egg yolk provides thirteen essential vitamins and minerals, including vitamins A, D, E, B12, riboflavin, folic acid, iron, zinc, and phosphorus. These nutrients have many functions, such as promoting good vision, maintaining healthy skin, improving resistance to infection, building healthy red blood cells, and maintaining the central nervous system—to name only a few! Egg yolk is the major source for the egg's vitamins and minerals, including vitamin D.[32, 33]

However, it is wise to consider only purchasing your eggs from farms where they allow the poultry out on pasture, rather than keeping them confined. For one thing, eggs from pastured poultry contain more nutrients. In 1974, a study published in the *British Journal of Nutrition* found that eggs from pastured hens had 50 percent more folic acid and 70 percent more vitamin B12 than eggs from factory-farmed hens.[34] In a study released in the *Journal of Agriculture and Food Chemistry*, eggs from hens raised on pasture were also found to be higher in lutein and zeaxanthin,[35] antioxidants that may help protect against macular degeneration, cancer, and cardiovascular disease. New research also shows that greater intake of lutein and zeaxanthin may reduce the risk of developing non-Hodgkin's lymphoma.[36]

Eggs from pastured chickens are also healthier in other ways. Salmonella infections are usually present only in traditionally raised commercial hens. Raw whole eggs are a phenomenally inexpensive and incredible source of high-quality nutrients that many people are deficient in, especially high-quality protein and fat. But many are afraid of raw eggs because they are worried about salmonella.

The risk of contracting salmonella from raw eggs is actually quite low. According to a study by the U.S. Department of Agriculture, only 0.003 percent of eggs—one in 30,000—are infected.[37] And if you are purchasing your eggs from healthy chickens, the infection risk is reduced even further. Remember, sick chickens are the ones most likely to lay salmonella-contaminated eggs.

If you are not used to fresh raw eggs you should start by eating just a tiny bit of it on a daily basis, and then gradually increase the portions. Fresh raw egg yolk tastes like vanilla and is best combined with vegetable pulp. You can also combine it with avocado. Only stir it gently with a fork, because egg protein easily gets damaged on a molecular level, even by mixing or blending. If you are so phenomenally unlucky as to come across an infected egg, a salmonella infection is typically not a major problem if you are healthy. You may feel sick and have loose stools, but this infection is easily treated by using large amounts of high-quality probiotics that have plenty of good bacteria. You can take a dose every thirty minutes until you start to feel better, and most people improve within a few hours.

The fact that eggs from pastured poultry are both more nutritious and less likely to be infected with disease is far from surprising, as foods that are produced naturally and organically are always much more likely to be healthy for you than processed, factory-farmed products laden with artificial chemicals and preservatives.

> "The main characteristic of Nature's farming can therefore be summed up in a few words. Mother earth never attempts to farm without livestock; she always raises mixed crops; great pains are taken to preserve the soil and to prevent erosion; the mixed vegetables and animals wastes are converted into humus; there is no waste; the processes of growth and the processes of decay balance one another; ample provision is made to maintain large reserves of fertility; the greatest care is taken to store the rainfall; both plants and animals are left to protect themselves against disease."
>
> —SIR ALBERT HOWARD, *An Agricultural Testament*[38]

Was Your Food Produced In a Foreign Country With Poor Inspection Standards?

A bill called C.O.O.L (Country of Origin Labeling) recently passed in Congress, but it is currently not being enforced due to lack of funding. One of its many initiatives requires a listing of the country of origin for beef, lamb, pork, fish, perishable agricultural commodities, and peanuts.[39] The large food corporations are threatened by this bill, because they worry that consumers will resist buying foods if they know where they've come from.

They're right to worry, and you should also be concerned. With companies like Wal-Mart entering the organic food market, it is very clear that much of our food supply will soon be grown outside the United States, where certification and inspection standards are not as stringent.

Some businesses are taking steps to support local food production. In June 2006, the organic retailer Whole Foods Market announced that it would commit $10 million to supporting locally grown food.[40] They will be making long-term, low-interest loans to small farms, especially producers of grass-fed beef and organic pasture-based eggs. They also announced that they would provide space in their parking lots to host open air markets for local farms. This is a welcome change, considering that Whole Foods Market has previously been criticized for compromising organic values—currently, for example, when you buy "organic" eggs, dairy, or meat at Whole Foods the animals may have been raised indoors rather than outside on pasture.[41]

Hopefully, Whole Foods Market's initiatives will pressure other large retailers to buy more locally produced foods and, at the same time, improve the current organic standards.

Also, in June 2006, the Pennsylvania Department of Agriculture launched an ad campaign called "Keep Pennsylvania Growing."[42] This campaign is designed to help consumers identify local products when they shop. If more states support this type of marketing, then we could see a growth in the number of local farms. Small farmers simply don't have the money to launch these types of initiatives on their own.

If you shop at the grocery store, ask your grocer where the food they sell was produced (not where it was packaged—companies often "cheat" by packaging their food closer at hand so they can pretend it's a domestic product). Better yet, buy your food directly from a local farm.

Even food that is genuinely organically produced can travel several thousand miles before it arrives at your local health food store or market, so purchasing from local farms decreases fuel transportation costs and reduces the time to your kitchen. More importantly, the only reliable way to ensure that your food has been produced using sound, organic, natural techniques is to visit the individual small farms and confirm that for yourself.

Do the Lower Prices of Global Trade
Justify the Negative Consequences?

You may not realize the consequences of the increase in global food trade. The current industrialized food system has obligated society to surrender to an "anonymous" food supply, which has dissociated us from the source of our food.

Between 1968 and 1998, world food trade increased 184 percent. The United States and many other industrialized nations are increasingly importing many of their foods from other countries. Increasing the reliance on imported foods means we also increase the transportation costs attached to our food, which results in the increased use of fossil fuels and contributes to global warming. In 1981, fresh produce arriving by truck at the Chicago Terminal Market traveled approximately 1,245 miles.[43] By 1998, that figure increased by 22 percent to 1,518 miles.[44]

COMPARISON OF LOCAL VERSUS CONVENTIONAL SOURCE FOOD MILES FOR PRODUCE[45]
WASD = WEIGHTED AVERAGE SOURCE DISTANCE

PRODUCT TYPE	LOCALLY GROWN WASD (MILES)	CONVENTIONAL SOURCE ESTIMATION WASD (MILES)
Apples	61	1,726
Beans	65	1,313
Broccoli	20	1,846
Cabbage	50	719
Carrots	27	1,838
Corn, Sweet	20	1,426
Garlic	31	1,811
Lettuce	43	1,823

Used with permission from the Leopold Center for Sustainable Agriculture

Onions	35	1,759
Peppers	44	1,589
Potatoes	75	1,155
Pumpkins	41	311
Spinach	36	1,815
Squash	52	1,277
Strawberries	56	1,830
Tomatoes	60	1,569
WASD (for all produce)	56	1,494
Sum of all WASDs	716	25,301

Conventional Food Travels Farther[46]

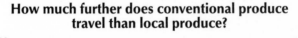

How much further does conventional produce travel than local produce?

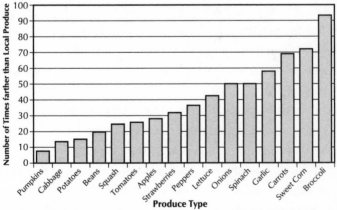

Used with permission from the Leopold Center for Sustainable Agriculture

Note: Local produce data from 2001 Practical Farmers of Iowa "All Iowa Meals."
Conventional source data derived by interpolating USDA AMS produce arrival data.

The above graph demonstrates just how many more miles are attached to foods that are not locally grown. Conventional broccoli traveled more than ninety times farther than locally grown broccoli;

carrots, sweet corn, garlic, onions, and spinach traveled at least fifty times farther.

Globalization has enabled the international food corporations to exploit less expensive human labor overseas. According to Bill Heffernan, professor emeritus of the University of Missouri, "About 21 percent of the world's population earns a dollar or less per day. Almost one-half of the world's population does not make over two dollars a day . . . If these people are going to be part of the global food system, it will most likely be as producers, not as consumers."[47]

In other words, for the transnational food corporations to increase their profits, they have been shifting to third world countries to produce food, rather than paying the higher costs of labor and land in the United States. While this has some beneficial economic effects, there are also inevitable consequences as a result of using this approach, which could far outweigh the reduced prices and increased profits.

The global trade system has indeed been highly effective at reducing the percentage of income that is actually spent on food. In an interview on the radio show *Beyond Organic* with host Jerry Kay, Michael Pollan, journalist and author of the book *The Omnivore's Dilemma: A Natural History of Four Meals*, explained that "today, Americans only spend about 9 percent of their income on food, which is very low. At the time I was a kid, in the 1960s', Americans spent about 20 percent of their income on food."[48]

But he also pointed out that as we have decreased the percentage of what we spend on food, the cost of health care has increased "from 5 percent to 16 percent."[49] The change in the food supply has had unquestionable direct correlations with the decline in your health. As I stated in the last chapter, many experts believe it is one of the primary reasons for the increase in nearly all chronic degenerative diseases, including our current epidemics of obesity, diabetes, Alzheimer's disease, and cancer.

Additionally, as more food is farmed abroad, less is grown domestically, so the global food trade has also contributed to the decline in farmers throughout North America. In 1960, there were approximately 15 million farmers in the United States. As a result of increased global trade, by 2000 this figure nose-dived to fewer than 2 million.[50]

Professor Heffernan warns that the actions of retailers like Wal-Mart will only worsen the situation for North American farmers. As they look to increase their profits while driving prices as low as possible, they will encourage the companies that produce the food they sell to turn to developing nations.

Wal-Mart is now the #1 organic food retailer in the United States. With the organic industry growing at a rate of about 20 percent per year, it's no surprise that they have decided to join in on a lucrative $15 billion market.[51] And with Wal-Mart's reputation for squeezing out its competitors, it will be interesting to see what happens to other popular natural health retailers such as Whole Foods or Wild Oats.

The important thing to keep in mind is that Wal-Mart wants to find the lowest priced suppliers. They will achieve this goal by outsourcing much of their food production to countries like China, where an entire province has been designated an "organic" food-growing area.[52] But remember that the definition of "organic" can be deceptive, and one reason the prices are lower abroad is not just because the cost of labor and land is less expensive, but also because rules are probably less stringent.

If you want to receive the maximum benefits of organic foods, make sure the food has been produced locally and that it hasn't been processed. If not, you will not only compromise your health, but you will be contributing to the loss of North American farmers. According to Heffernan, "Wal-Mart will contribute to the further decline in the number of our farmers. The only way to stop this trend is for consumers to buy food from local farmers."[53] He warns consumers that, in an extreme example, if they don't change where they shop, we could wake up one day to find that all of our farmers are gone.

> "Economists . . . have never bothered to place a value on the lives of farm families that have been destroyed by the loss of their farms, their way of life, and their heritage. They have never bothered to consider the value of the lives of rural people—with roots in rural schools, churches, and businesses—who were forced to abandon their communities as farm families were forced off the land."
>
> —JOHN IKERD,
> Professor Emeritus, University of Missouri[54]

Why Should You Buy Local Food?

As people have learned about the consequences of factory farming and global trade, many have gradually shifted their shopping habits, choosing to purchase large portions of their food from farmers' markets and CSA's (Community-Supported Agriculture operations).

CSA's are a relatively recent phenomenon in food production. They are based on the idea of small-scale organic farmers selling their produce to local area residents. The decreased food transportation charges and higher quality of the food provide exceptional value for those who use this system. Normally, individuals pay a membership fee to join a local CSA, which entitles them to buy an array of organically produced foods (vegetables, fruits, herbs, milk, and meat products). Some CSA's focus on a system of weekly delivery or pick-up.

There are many reasons to patronize CSA's, as well as farmers' markets, family farms, and other small, sustainable food producers. Doing so:

1. Avoids pesticides, genetically modified foods, hormones, and antibiotics

2. Improves food safety and security

3. Protects future generations

4. Increases biodiversity

5. Improves ecological harmony (preserves the environment, less erosion, increased water quality)

6. Provides fresh, wholesome food with better taste and nutrition

7. Decreases the use of fossil fuels (reduces global warming)

8. Supports the ethical treatment of animals

9. Saves farming heritage

10. Improves rural economy

Typically, small family farms focus much of their attention on the quality of the food they produce and work hard to protect the environment. Rather than continuously confining their animals, they allow their animals to graze on pasture, which helps to improve the health of the animals, as well as increasing the amount of nutrition in their meat.

Putting animals on pasture dramatically decreases the risk of contaminating local water supplies, and helps fertilize and build the topsoil. Many small farmers practice methods that improve the quality of the soil, ensuring the sustainability of future high-quality food harvests. These farmers understand that high-quality soil also equates to higher-quality food. One final important benefit is that food raised with these methods typically taste much better than food purchased in conventional grocery stores. And isn't that one of the primary purposes of food—to taste good?

Preserving the Topsoil Helps
Preserve Your Health

One serious consequence of raising animals in confinement operations is the loss of precious topsoil. When the animals are out to pasture, rather than confined, they naturally fertilize and rebuild the topsoil which is critical to nourishing healthy plants.

Eatwild.com outlines the differences in soil erosion based upon the various methods used to feed animals. Since the United States is losing three billion tons of nutrient-rich topsoil each year, it is important for agriculturalists to develop strategies which emphasize building rather than reducing topsoil.[55] Animals in feedlots are fed high amounts of corn and soy. Growing corn and soy for animal feed contributes to the reduction of topsoil, whereas pasture reduces soil loss by as much as 93 percent.

Pasture Reduces Topsoil Erosion By
93 Percent[56]

Soil Erosion

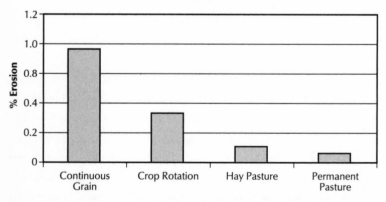

Chart courtesy of Jo Robinson (http://www.eatwild.com/ReadMore13.htm)
Source: Control of Soil Erosion: Ontario Ministry of Agriculture and Food, Robert P. Stone and Neil Moore (1996) http://www.omatra.gov.on.ca/englis/engineer/facts/95-089.htm[57]

4[""]

The next graph shows the results of a study conducted by the University of Wisconsin Discovery Farms Program, which revealed that, compared with grazed pasture, gently sloped land devoted to soy and corn production lost six times more topsoil each year. According to Dennis Frame, the director of Discovery Farms, if the trend of selling cows and moving to grain production doesn't cease, soil erosion and nutrient losses will continue to climb.[58]

Growing Corn and Soy Causes Six Times More Soil Erosion Than Pasture[59]

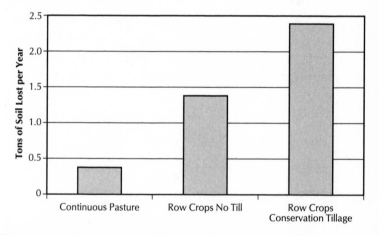

Chart courtesy of Jo Robinson http://www.eatwild.com/ReadMore10.htm
Based upon "The Role Of The Dairy Industry In Protecting Surface Water Quality",
University of Wisconsin—Discovery Farms Program
http://www.discoveryfarms.org/special/other/roledairy.pdf.

Choosing Local Farms for Your Foods

Familiarizing yourself with whoever is producing your food is an important factor in obtaining the highest quality food possible. Local farmers can be asked what techniques and strategies they use to produce their food. If you visit the farm or CSA, you can actually see for yourself which agricultural practices are being employed. If you're concerned about whether or not the animals are out on pasture, for example, you can drive to the farm and take a look.

Ask farmers specific questions about whether they use antibiotics, hormones, fertilizers or pesticides and, more times than not, they'll be happy to tell you just how they produce their food.

If they are unwilling to have this discussion, then it would be better for you to find another farmer that will. If you're confused about where to find local farmers, one good place to start is the farmers' market. The good news is that the number of farmers' markets in the United States doubled between 1994 and 2004.[60]

Farmers' Market Growth, 1994-2004[61]

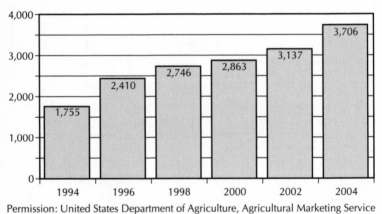

Operating Markets

Permission: United States Department of Agriculture, Agricultural Marketing Service

Traditionally, farmers' markets have been available for consumers to meet the producers of the foods they buy. However, sometimes it can be hit and miss. It is not uncommon to buy food at farmers markets that is sold by "vendors" rather than the actual producers. And if they are a vendor, they may have simply bought the produce at the local food depot (where the food can come in from long distances) rather than from a local farm. So don't be fooled; be sure to ask the person standing at the food stand if they are a farmer or a vendor and if you're talking to a vendor, simply ask to make sure they are selling food from local sources.

If you're interested in finding a farmers' market in your area, the USDA has created the National Directory of Farmers Markets, which is available online at: www.ams.usda.gov/farmersmarkets/map.htm

Unfortunately, locally produced foods are still only a small fraction of the $900 billion U.S. food industry. But according to Bob Pierson, director of local food advocacy groups Food Trust and Farm to City, consumer spending on locally produced food has grown dramatically: "Sales at farmers' markets and other ventures coordinated by Farm to City have climbed from less than $200,000 in 2001 to $625,000 last year."[62] Ann Karlen, director of Fair Food Farmstead in Philadelphia's Reading Terminal Market, reported that spending there increased from $88,000 in 2004 to $123,275 in 2005.[63]

After learning about the unethical and disease-promoting agricultural practices occurring within the poultry industry, you may be happy to learn that there are numerous local small farms producing pastured poultry. In a pastured setting, the chickens are exposed to sunlight and graze on grass, bugs and weeds.

Brian Moyer is a board member of the American Pastured Poultry Producers Association (APPPA), and the owner and operator of Green Haven Farm in Berks County, Pennsylvania. Green Haven markets their chickens, eggs, lamb and goat cheese through two CSA's, two farmers' markets, restaurants and direct-on-the-farm sales.

Increasingly, Moyer is noticing that consumers are choosing pastured poultry over commercial sources: "Consumers want pastured poultry. They are starting to question how factory chickens are produced. When they choose a pastured chicken or egg, they feel that they are making a healthier choice. Plus, they prefer the taste."[64] He notes that there is a particular increase in demand for locally produced food among couples in their 30s who have young children.

Bird Flu Would Never Exist If All Chickens Were Raised This Way

Joel Salatin of Polyface Farm in Virginia, who you might recall from Chapter 4, has been involved in the raising of pastured poultry for 40 years. Salatin actually raises six different animals for food—cattle, chickens, turkeys, pigs, rabbits and sheep. He refers to his poultry's diet as a "salad bar" as they graze on his plush pasture. His animals are thriving very well on their "salad bar" diet, and his chickens are extraordinarily healthy.

Recently, Salatin spoke with a federal inspector who had examined his chickens for an out-of-state sale. The inspector works with facilities that process poultry from "vertically integrated" operations—in other words, factory farming. During their conversation, the federal inspector told Salatin that his "worst chicken was better than the best chicken" coming from the factory farms.[65]

Salatin explains that you can tell the health of his chicken by examining the color of the liver, overall vibrancy of the organs, cleanliness around joints (which hold infection) as well as other markers. It's clear that Salatin is very proud of what he has developed in Polyface Farms. People travel for miles to visit his farm and buy the food he produces, and also to learn about how to raise pastured chickens.

In order to find out just how sanitary his chickens were, Salatin had his poultry tested. He had his chickens cultured for exterior bacteria in a laboratory that measured the results in colony forming units (cfu) per milliliter to the second permutation. For comparison, the laboratory also cultured supermarket chickens.

The supermarket chicken averaged 3,600 cfu/ml and Salatin's chicken averaged 133 cfu/ml.[66] His chicken was 25 times "cleaner"—

that is to say, it had 25 times less colony forming units of bacteria—than the supermarket chicken.[67]

Choosing healthier poultry that are thriving, disease-free animals will go a lot further towards improving and maintaining your health than the commonly selected factory farmed alternative.

> **The multinational food corporations that increasingly control agriculture are not people—they have no heart, no soul, nor citizenship in any particular country. They will produce or buy agricultural commodities wherever they can produce or buy at the lowest cost, without regard for national origin. Our continuing quest for cheap food could mean the end of American agriculture.**
>
> **—JOHN IKERD,**
> **Professor Emeritus University of Missouri[68]**

More Chefs are Connecting with Local Farms

Many different people and groups are starting to realize the importance of purchasing their food from local farms. Chefs like Tod Murphy, founder of The Farmer's Diner in Barre, Vermont, spends about 65 cents of every food dollar on locally produced foods.[69] When asked if Vermont could feed itself one day, he replied, "Vermont citizens/farmers could produce about 70–85 percent of the calories we consume as a state. To get from where we are today to that would take about six years and a substantial financial investment.[70]

"The issue would be the people. Right now there are roughly 6,500 farms here. We would need about 60,000 to 100,000 farms and processors of various sizes to meet the needs of 650,000 residents.

This combined with becoming energy-independent are the two most worthy objectives of government and citizens."[71]

Murphy clearly understands the importance of teamwork. If we expect to solve the problems inherent in our food supply today, we will all have to work together to support local farmers.

Celebrity Chef Rick Bayless (www.fronterakitchens.com) of Chicago also recognizes the importance of supporting local farms. Every year, he buys plenty of his food locally, including thousands of pounds of tomatoes to make his famous salsa. He says his customers notice a difference in taste, which keeps them coming back for more.

The Chefs Collaborative (www.chefscollaborative.org), the Slow Food association (www.slowfood.com), and the Weston A. Price Foundation (www.westonaprice.org) are other organizations involved in connecting consumers to farmers (see the resource section in the Appendix or go to www.mercola.com for a more comprehensive list). The movement toward reviving farming communities is gaining a great deal of momentum. Alternative Farming Systems Information Center also provides the names of many groups helping in the effort to build sustainable agriculture.[72]

The Bright Side of Local Agriculture

One such organization is the Food Circles Networking Project at the University of Missouri-Columbia founded by Professors Bill Heffernan and Mary Hendrickson.[73] The goal of the project is to develop a community-based, sustainable food system. Borrrowed from Green Philosophy arguments made by the Kansas City Food Circle, their philosophy is built on four fundamental principles:

Ecological Wisdom:

Our food should be grown, shipped and eaten in a manner that respects the Earth's resources and protects the environment for ourselves and future generations.

Social Justice:

The farmers and workers who grow and process our food deserve a fair return for their labor. Every member of a community should have access to healthy, wholesome food regardless of income.

Grassroots Democracy:

Control over our food should rest with us. Decisions about who grows our food, where and how it is grown, and who gets to eat should not be left with transnational corporations but rather should be up to communities and the people in those communities.

Non-violence:

The animals who provide us food and fiber should be treated humanely, just as the farmers and laborers who grow and process our food should be treated with respect and dignity.[74]

Unfortunately, for several decades now, most of our universities have been teaching and promoting industrial agriculture. But some universities have started innovative new farming programs in an attempt to create healthier, more sustainable agricultural practices. The Leopold Center for Sustainable Agriculture at Iowa State University is a research and education center with statewide programs to develop agricultural practices that are both profitable and conserve natural resources.[75] It was established under the Groundwater Protection Act of 1987.

Ohio State University Extension in Athens, Ohio, is also

studying the benefits of sustainable agricultural practices, such as grazing.[76] Through the Appalachian Farming Systems Research Center (AFSRC) in West Virginia, the USDA is examining the agricultural practices of small family farms.[77]

Stop Factory Farms Before It's Too Late

On January 9, 2004, the Johns Hopkins Bloomberg School of Public Health issued a press release demanding a moratorium on the building of new CAFOs. The American Public Health Association (APHA) cited a number of problems with CAFOs, including:

- The contamination of drinking water with pathogens from animal waste runoff
- Growing antibiotic resistance resulting from the millions of pounds of antibiotics routinely fed to animals
- Severe respiratory problems in CAFO workers
- Illnesses among people living near CAFO operations[78]

Robert Lawrence, MD, director of the Center for a Livable Future, is in agreement with this moratorium. According to Lawrence, "Factory farms make their workers sick, pollute the environment, and pose serious public health risks to people living nearby."[79]

After reading through this list of concerns described by Johns Hopkins, one is left to wonder how CAFOs were ever approved by any government agency in the first place.

Fifty-four percent of livestock in the United States are now confined to just 5 percent of livestock farms. These CAFOs generate 575 billion pounds of animal waste each year, contaminated with salmonella, campylobacter, cryptosporidium, E. coli, heavy metals, nitrogen, phosphorus, and an estimated 13 million pounds of antibiotics. These billions of pounds of animal waste are frequently stored on floodplains on alluvial aquifers, contaminating drinking water supplies.[80]

In addition, as was mentioned in chapter 3, many studies of CAFOs have documented respiratory problems in workers, including chronic bronchitis and nonallergic asthma. Workers at CAFOs are also exposed to the potent neurotoxin hydrogen sulfide, and studies of people living near CAFOs describe eye and respiratory symptoms. And the routine feeding of antibiotics to animals in CAFOs is also helping fuel the growing problem of antibiotic resistant pathogens, not just among CAFO employees but in the entire population.[81]

As if that weren't enough, CAFOs are also notoriously inhumane to animals. Life for an animal in a factory farm is one of acute deprivation, stress, and disease. Farm animals are forced to live in cages just barely larger than their own bodies and usually spend their entire lives without seeing daylight.[82]

Before the collusion between the media and the corporations, producing healthy food was the priority in every society. Historically, man used common sense to produce and choose his foods wisely. Now, most of us are choosing to avoid giving any serious thought as to how our food has been produced or how it will nourish us.

Officials who claim that factory farmed food is safe, and small local farms are responsible for spreading bird flu, are the same "experts" who approved spraying DDT on crops, irradiating your food, and planting untested genetically engineered crops.

We need to stop blindly accepting the credibility of the "experts" who approve of practices that are detrimental to your health. If they were truly experts, they would be encouraging and promoting small, local, organic farms, rather than the hellish factory farms that have become the standard source of your food.

It is the intention of this book to create an awareness of the dangerous and inhumane practices that appear to be the true cause of the bird flu threat. If enough attention can be drawn to these serious issues, then the corporations that run those farms and their allies in the media and government will have made a serious strategic error by crying wolf about the relatively minor problem of bird flu.

Their apparent attempt to instill fear in the population, presumably in order to drive their competitors out of business, will instead result in increased knowledge of a main cause of the spread of bird flu—their own highly questionable practices.

> **"The human costs of cheap food have been undeniably tremendous, but since they couldn't be measured in dollars and cents, they have gone uncounted."**
>
> **—JOHN IKERD,**
> **Professor Emeritus, University of Missouri[83]**

Avian Flu—The Truth
A guest commentary by Joel Salatin

At our farm here in Virginia's Shenandoah Valley we've raised outdoor pastured poultry for nearly half a century without a single case of avian flu. During that time, it has struck industrial confinement birds in our area several times, the last being in 2002 when 1,000 tractor trailer loads of birds were land filled, incinerated, or buried on site (all this known euphemistically as "depopulation") and then indemnified with taxpayer money.

International monitoring think-tank GRAIN has identified industrial poultry import-export trade routes as the primary vector for spreading this disease. This global traf-ficking includes chicken guts, feathers, eggs, chicks, and edible product. So far, every outbreak in the world has occurred in industrial poultry production centers. The outbreak in India resulted in half a million birds being destroyed in a 1.5 mile radius of the outbreak—that's roughly 25 Tyson-style factory houses in a 1.5 mile radius.

While migratory birds may carry some of the virus, it quickly dissipates in areas where industrial confinement facilities do not exist. In a recent report, James Roth, Iowa State University veterinarian and researcher, identified U.S. animal agriculture as being the sector most vulnerable to pathogens and listed the first four reasons as:

- High-density animal husbandry

- The high rate of transportation and mingling of animals

- No immunity in U.S. herds and flocks to foreign animal diseases; no vaccinations for such diseases

- Centralized feed supplies and distribution channels[84]

What would a production system without these vul-nerabilities look like? Birds would be diffused around the countryside in smaller flocks; production, processing, and marketing would be local events with community commerce; production models would encourage immune systems in domestic flocks; feed sources would be bio-regional rather than global. This is exactly what our farm and thousands of pastured poultry producers around the world practice.

And yet we are demonized by the global industrial establishment as being perpetrators of pathogenicity because our birds commune with red-winged blackbirds. New United States Department of Agriculture research discovered a high number of farm ponds that attract waterfowl. Researchers found this "shocking" because it may entice bird flu. For decades, farmers have been encouraged, through both government and private programs, to protect riparian areas and to respect the water resource. Suddenly this wonderful asset—water—is being demonized as a liability.

The chickens and turkeys on our farm have a heightened immune system because they interact with their environment. Their numbers are consistent with ecological carrying capacity, both on our farm and in the bioregion. They are processed right on the farm, not trucked up the interstate to seed the countryside with millions of pathogen-laden feathers. They are not comingled with birds from other farms, and we don't feed dead chickens to our chickens.

Everything in nature marks boundaries. Dogs mark their turf. Deer mark their turf. Cell walls protect their interior from foreign invasion. Fences are not all bad. They keep our children in the yard or protect them from the swimming pool. As a culture, the transnational global agenda of a food system without barriers carries inherent risks. And recently USDA secretary Mike Johanns disclosed plans to ship whole broilers to China, hotbed of

SARS and avian flu, to be processed and shipped back to the United States for domestic consumption.

Biological things become acclimated to their place; putting down roots is a healthy thing. Those of us dedicated to producing, processing, and marketing in our foodscapes offer a completely different paradigm to the industrial confinement global factory fare. The only threat we present is a healthy alternative and real remedies for their problems. On our farm, we are much more concerned about the industrial-bureaucratic response to avian flu when it arrives again, like it has many times, than we are about the vulnerability of our own domestic pastured birds.

The fraternity of experts analyzing and pontificating about avian flu is the same club that told us farmers to feed dead cows to our cows, to sprinkle DDT over everything, to use petroleum-based chemical fertilizers because manure wasn't worth hauling to the fields, and to "get big or get out." Their track record is dismal.

> **The fraternity of experts analyzing and pontificating about avian flu is the same club that told us farmers to feed dead cows to our cows, to sprinkle DDT over everything, to use petroleum-based chemical fertilizers because manure wasn't worth hauling to the fields, and to "get big or get out." Their track record is dismal.**

Each of us knows that when we crowd children in a room, we're going to have sickness. And the longer they're crowded in that room, the more sickness we'll have. Compound that a thousand-fold, and you have the pattern of modern industrial confinement animal agriculture. Predicated on Neanderthal science, Concentrated Animal Feeding Operations (CAFOs) are monuments to the stupidity of man. Every paradigm exceeds its point of efficiency. Food is primarily biology, not industry.

Avian flu is just one example of nature speaking, indeed screaming, "Enough!" But the industrialist is too busy counting money and pouring concrete and smelting iron to listen. Are you? Am I?

8

RESOURCES AND ORGANIZATIONS TO HELP YOU STAY INFORMED

You are continuously deluged with media messages. Every day, the average American is exposed to about 3,000 advertising messages alone.[1]

The media provides important and vital information about the world you live in. But much of this information is simply distorted hyperbole or misleading deceptions designed to control your behavior. Powerful corporate interests have a vested interest in making sure that you only hear the messages that they want you to hear.

The bird flu pandemic is merely another media-manufactured subterfuge among many. There have been similar, previous attempts to frighten you—from swine flu to West Nile virus to SARS—and you can be virtually assured that there will be future attempts to manipulate your behavior.

It appears that the international corporate poultry operations hope that their apparent bird flu strategy will provide the leverage they need to help them regulate their competitors out of business. The drug manufacturers have used it as an excuse to obtain billions of dollars of federal subsidies, and to sell billions of dollars worth of ineffective and potentially toxic drugs. These marketing geniuses will use every trick they can to help increase their bottom lines.

One of the major corporate goals is to increase your use of their products. So you are routinely fed carefully planned deceptions about how best to take care of your health, what food to purchase, and what agricultural techniques are sustainable and sound. You are regularly exposed to biased science, contrived news reports, and sophisticated corporate-sponsored media pieces that are presented as "news."

To help you sort through this complex distortions of reality, I founded a Web site ten years ago, www.mercola.com, that is dedicated to that purpose, but there certainly are other powerful sources of information that will help you understand the truth.

Here are three simple principles that you can use to help you in your journey to sort though the corporate deceptions:

- Follow the money. Always find out who is paying for a study or funding a foundation.

- If something doesn't make sense to you, start asking some questions. In the matter of your health, learn what illnesses are truly dangerous and what their actual causes are; where and how your food was produced; what agricultural practices are truly sustainable and prevent the spread of disease; and what activities and lifestyle habits are and aren't healthy for you.

- Be a personal witness. If there is an important issue, examine the evidence yourself. For one example, you can buy your food from a place where you can have a look at how it was grown or raised.

For those of you who don't have the time to do your own research, you will have to rely on (hopefully) objective reporters or informed intermediaries to tell the truth. But there's no need for you to try to spot the deceptions all on your own. There are many genuinely independent groups and organizations searching for the truth. This chapter is intended to help identify a few that I am personally aware of. However, if you know of any that are not here, please go to our Web site: www.GreatBirdFluHoax.com, and send us an e-mail with ones you have found helpful.

RSS News Feeds—Your Key to Tapping Into the Information Network

My staff and I sort through many hundreds of articles every day to find out what the latest news is. We do this inexpensively thanks to the Internet and the relatively recent technology of RSS news feeds. RSS stands for Real Simple Syndication, and it is a technology that allows Web sites to automatically update your computer with the latest stories as they break. RSS feeds can help you stay informed on bird flu and other matters of importance, giving you news from a variety of sources so that you can read more than one perspective. Other resources we list later in the chapter can help you sort through them and separate the real news from the propaganda.

There are tens of thousands of Web sites that have these feeds (including Mercola.com). The new version of Microsoft Internet Explorer version 7, which will be officially launched in early 2007, will allow you to easily add RSS feeds to your browser. The Firefox browser allows you to do that right now.

I personally have used a stand-alone application called SharpReader (www.sharpreader.net) for the last four years to access over 10,000 stories a month. The beauty of RSS news feeds is that you can get as little or as many articles as you want, on just about any subject that your heart desires.

Once you have installed an RSS news feed aggregator, either a stand-alone version like SharpReader, or a browser-based one like

Firefox or Internet Explorer version 7, then you can fill up your reader with RSS news feeds.

Here are a few sites you can go to in order to search different feeds:

RADIO USER LAND TOP 100 MOST SUBSCRIBED FEEDS
radio.xmlstoragesystem.com/rcsPublic/rssHotlist

BLOGLINES TOP FEEDS
www.bloglines.com/topblogs

THOUSANDS MORE TO CHOOSE FROM
www.rss-network.com

How to Protect Yourself Against the Evil Marketing Geniuses

If you found this book helpful, and want to remain informed about many similar health issues, be sure to subscribe to the free health newsletter at Mercola.com. In the fall of 2006, the Web site plans on implementing an innovative Web 2.0 section that will allow you to participate in the development of a system to help identify health truths and deceptions.

There are other organizations that exist to make sure that the news and information you get is either accurate, or correctly identified as deceptive. News in the mainstream media is no longer news, so it is important to find alternative views on various stories if we expect to even come close to finding out the truth.

Resources to Help You Sort Through the Media

There are many independent media sources on the Internet that are acting as "watchdogs" over mainstream media, because they have a great deal to cover. We are NOT receiving the fair and balanced news we all deserve to hear or read about. It would be difficult to list all of the independent news services available (apologies to those I missed), but here are a few:

Center for Media and Democracy
www.prwatch.org

The Center for Media and Democracy promotes a democratic media and exposes public relations spin and propaganda.

Fairness and Accuracy in reporting (FAIR)
www.fair.org

FAIR is a national media watch group that is very critical of media bias and censorship. Their goal is to advocate for greater diversity in the press by exposing stories that would not be reported in mainstream media. FAIR supports the need to expand the media by breaking up the dominant media conglomerates and strengthening independent media.

Rocky Mountain Media Watch
www.bigmedia.org

Rocky Mountain Media Watch is seeking to create better news for a strong democracy. They want to heighten the public's awareness about just how "Big Media" manipulates its viewers. Their goal is to offer better, more democratic journalism.

AlterNet
www.alternet.org

AlterNet is an online community that offers original journalism and carries news from several other independent media sources. AlterNet wants to inspire citizen action and advocacy by focusing on stories about the environment, human rights and civil liberties, social justice, media, and health care issues.

Accuracy in Media (AIM)
www.aim.org

Accuracy in Media is a nonprofit, grassroots citizens' watchdog of the news media whose purpose is to set the record straight on stories that have received biased coverage.

Other Resources

Below you will find a list of organizations concerned with the issues of health, diet, animal welfare, the environment, and sustainable agriculture raised in this book. There are far too many groups to mention here (apologies to those I missed). In addition to these organizations, be sure to find local sustainable agricultural groups in your area; many of them hold extremely informative annual meetings where you can meet local farmers.

- If you are concerned about the quality of the food you are buying at the grocery store, some of the following links will help guide you to healthier, more humane choices through local farms.

- If you are interested in stopping factory farming, some of the following links will help show you how to get involved.

- If you are a farmer who is interested in producing healthy and ecologically sustainable food, there are links below that will help show you how.

- Some of the following links will provide you with scientific literature supporting the benefits of sustainable agriculture.

Information about Factory Farming

The Meatrix
www.themeatrix.com

An entertaining video animation about factory farming and links about what you can do about it.

Beyond Factory Farming
www.beyondfactoryfarming.org

Beyond Factory Farming is a coalition of citizen's organizations from all across Canada. Their goal is to promote livestock production that supports food sovereignty and sustainability, and ecological, human, and animal health.

Wegmans Cruelty
www.wegmanscruelty.com

A video showing what goes on inside a factory chicken farm. The site also includes news related to factory farming.

Information about Healthy Food

Weston A. Price Foundation
www.westonaprice.org

The goal of the Weston A. Price Foundation is to restore nutrient-dense traditional foods to the human diet through education, research, and activism. In order to achieve their goal, the foundation supports accurate nutrition instruction, organic and biodynamic farming, pasture feeding of livestock, and community-supported farms.

Price-Pottenger Nutrition Foundation
www.price-pottenger.org

> The Price-Pottenger Nutrition Foundation, a nonprofit educational organization, is a clearinghouse of information on healthful lifestyles, ecology, sound nutrition, alternative medicine, humane farming, and organic gardening.

Slow Food
www.slowfood.com

> The association's activities seek to defend biodiversity in the food supply, educate people regarding the importance of taste, and link producers of excellent foods to consumers through events and initiatives.

Sustainable Table
www.sustainabletable.org

> Sustainable Table promotes and educates consumers about making healthy food choices that support a sustainable system.

The Community Food Security Coalition (CFSC)
www.foodsecurity.org

> CFSC is a North American organization dedicated to building strong, sustainable, local and regional food systems that ensure access to affordable, nutritious, and culturally appropriate food.

Organic Consumers Association (OCA)
www.organicconsumers.org

> OCA is building a national network of consumers promoting issues such as food safety, organic agriculture, fair trade, and sustainability.

The True Food Network
www.truefoodnow.org

> The goal of the True Food Network is to create a socially just, democratic, and sustainable food system.

Access to Healthy Food

Local Harvest
www.localharvest.org

> This Web site will help you find farmers' markets, family farms, and other sources of sustainably grown food in your area, where you can buy produce, grass-fed meats, and many other goodies.

Farmers' Markets
www.ams.usda.gov/farmersmarkets

> A national listing of farmers' markets.

Eat Wild
www.eatwild.com

> Eatwild.com is an excellent source for safe, healthy, natural, and nutritious grass-fed beef, lamb, goats, bison, poultry, pork, and dairy products.

Eat Well Guide: Wholesome Food from Healthy Animals
www.eatwellguide.org/About.cfm

> The Eat Well Guide is a free online directory of sustainably raised meat, poultry, dairy, and eggs from farms, stores, restaurants, inns, and hotels, and online outlets in the United States and Canada.

FoodRoutes
www.foodroutes.org

> The FoodRoutes Find Good Food map can help you connect with local farmers so that you can find the freshest, tastiest food possible. On their interactive map, you can find a listing for local farmers, CSA's, and markets near you.

Food Circles
www.foodcircles.missouri.edu.
www.foodandsocietyfellows.org

> The goal of the project is to develop a community-based, sustainable food system.

Chefs Collaborative
www.chefscollaborative.org

> Chefs Collaborative is a national network promoting sustainable cuisine by supporting local, seasonal, and artisanal cooking.

Getting Healthy Foods Into the Schools

National Farm to School
www.farmtoschool.org

> Farm to School programs are becoming increasingly popular all over the United States. These programs connect schools with local farms in order to provide healthy meals in school cafeterias, improve student nutrition, and support local small farmers.

Farm to College
www.farmtocollege.org

> This site offers information about farm-to-college programs throughout North America collected by the Community Food Security Coalition.

Sustainable Food In Schools
www.sustainabletable.org/schools/dining

> If you don't like the food being served in your or your child's cafeteria, you can do something about it. This site includes guidelines on what to do, how to do it, and examples of successful efforts that have already been initiated in the United States.

> ## The Battle Against Genetically Modified (GM) Foods

Institute of Science in Society (ISIS)
www.i-sis.org.uk

> ISIS promotes responsible science, independent of commercial and other special interests, or of government control. ISIS advocates sustainability and promotes critical public understanding of the science of and debate over genetic modification.

EcoNexus
www.econexus.info

> EcoNexus is a public interest research organization and science watchdog. One of their goals is to investigate the impacts of genetic engineering on the environment, health, food security, agriculture, human rights, and society.

The Campaign
www.thecampaign.org

> The Campaign is creating a national grassroots consumer effort for the purpose of lobbying Congress and the president to pass legislation that will require the labeling of genetically engineered foods in the United States.

The Future of Food
www.thefutureoffood.com

> This is an excellent movie by Deborah Koons Garcia about the subject of genetic engineering.

GEAN (Genetic Engineering Action Network)
www.geaction.org

> GEAN USA is a support system for groups that are addressing the risks of genetic engineering.

Institute for Responsible Technology (IRT)
www.responsibletechnology.org

> The IRT promotes the responsible use of technology and is helping create strategies to stop genetically engineered foods and crops.

Ban Terminator
www.banterminator.org

> Terminators, or GURTS (Genetic Use Restriction Technologies), are a class of genetic engineering technologies that allow companies to introduce seeds whose sterile offspring cannot reproduce, preventing farmers from replanting seeds from their harvest. This genetic technology will give further control to a few corporate interests and will threaten the livelihoods of our farmers. Ban Terminator is working to stop this technology from entering our food supply.

The Non-GMO Report
www.non-gmoreport.com

> The Non-GMO Report provides information to help inform you about genetic engineering and help you find non-genetically modified products.

Council of Canadians
www.canadians.org

The Council of Canadians is active in promoting the GE-Free Canada Campaign and other important environmental issues.

Science and Research

Institute of Science in Society
www.i-sis.org.uk

(See listing in "The Battle Against Genetically Modified Foods" section.)

Union of Concerned Scientists (USC)
www.ucsusa.org

UCS is an independent nonprofit alliance of more than 100,000 concerned citizens and scientists working to build a cleaner, healthier environment and a safer world.

Organic Center for Education and Promotion (OCEP)
www.organic-center.org

The goal of OCEP is to generate credible, peer reviewed scientific information that illustrates the verifiable benefits of organic farming.

Sustainable Agriculture

Acres USA
www.acresusa.com

Acres USA offers a publication, Web site, and annual conference that support and educate farmers and consumers about sustainable agriculture.

National Sustainable Agriculture Information Service (ATTRA)
www.attra.ncat.org
> ATTRA provides information and technical assistance to farmers, ranchers, extension agents, educators, and others involved in sustainable agriculture.

Community Involved in Sustaining Agriculture (CISA)
www.buylocalfood.com
> CISA is dedicated to sustaining agriculture and promoting the products of small farms.

The Center for Food Safety (CFS)
www.centerforfoodsafety.org
> The (CFS) is working to legally challenge harmful food production technologies and promote sustainable alternatives.

Bioneers
www.bioneers.org
> Bioneers is working to develop programs that support conservation of biological and cultural diversity, traditional farming practices, and environmental restoration.

GRAIN
www.grain.org
> GRAIN is an international nongovernmental organization (NGO) that promotes agricultural sustainability and biodiversity.

Ecological Farming Association
www.eco-farm.org
> Eco-Farm is working to support the strengthening of the soil, the protection of the air and water, and diverse ecosystems and economies.

Kerr Center for Sustainable Agriculture
www.kerrcenter.com

> The Kerr Center provides farmers and ranchers with information about how to improve their operations.

National Campaign for Sustainable Agriculture
www.sustainableagriculture.net

> The National Campaign for Sustainable Agriculture is a diverse partnership of individuals and organizations supporting environmentally sound, profitable, healthy, humane and just food and agricultural systems.

Sustainable Agriculture Research and Education (SARE)
www.sare.org

> The SARE program supports sustainable farming systems through a nationwide research and education grants program.

Leopold Center for Sustainable Agriculture
www.leopold.iastate.edu

> The Leopold Center for Sustainable Agriculture explores and cultivates alternatives that are healthy for people and the environment.

Organizations for Independent and Family Farmers

National Farmers Union
www.nfu.org

> National Farmers Union is working to protect and enhance the economic well-being and quality of life for family farmers and ranchers and their rural communities. They believe that

consumers and producers can work together to promote local, safe food.

Family Farm Defenders
www.familyfarmdefenders.org

The goal of Family Farm Defenders is to support the rights of small farmers.

Institute for Agriculture and Trade Policy
www.iatp.org / www.sustain.org

The Institute for Agriculture and Trade Policy promotes family farms, rural communities, and ecosystems through research and education, science and technology, and advocacy.

Farm and Ranch Freedom Alliance
www.farmandranchfreedom.org

The Farm and Ranch Freedom Alliance is an advocate for the many thousands of independent farmers, ranchers, livestock owners, and homesteaders in the United States.

National Family Farm Coalition (NFFC)
www.nffc.net

The NFFC works to ensure fair prices for family farmers and promote safe and healthy food around the world.

Rural Coalition
www.ruralco.org

The Rural Coalition is an alliance of regionally and culturally diverse organizations working to build a more just and sustainable food system.

Important Physician Groups

American College for Advancement in Medicine (ACAM)

www.acam.org

ACAM is a not-for-profit medical society dedicated to educating health care professionals about the most current research in preventive/nutritional medicine.

American Holistic Medical Association (AHMA)

www.holisticmedicine.org

The AHMA was founded in 1978 as a membership organization for physicians seeking to practice a broader form of medicine than what has been and is currently being taught in allopathic (MD and DO) medical schools. AHMA educates physicians who are integrating holistic principles into their practice. Their membership of approximately one thousand professional health care practitioners is working to make the holistic model more widely available.

Association of American Physicians and Surgeons (AAPS)

www.aapsonline.org

AAPS is a national association of physicians dedicated to preserving freedom in the one-on-one patient-physician relationship. Its members believe this patient-physician relationship must be protected from all forms of third-party intervention. Since its founding in 1943, AAPS has been the only national organization consistently supporting the principles of the free market in medical practice.

American Association for Health Freedom (AAHF)
www.healthfreedom.net

> AAHF was founded in 1992 in direct response to the problems faced by health care practitioners and consumers in the United States. AAHF works as an advocate to restore the medical freedoms that have been threatened by the U.S. Food and Drug Administration, the allopathic medical community, insurance companies, and state medical boards around the United States.

American Academy of Environmental Medicine
www.aaem.com

> AAEM was founded in 1965, and is an international association of physicians and other professionals interested in the clinical aspects of man and his environment. The Academy is interested in expanding the knowledge of interactions between human individuals and their environment, as these may be demonstrated to be reflected in their total health.

Environmental Issues

Environmental Working Group (EWG)
www.ewg.org

> EWG specializes in environmental investigations. They have a team of scientists, engineers, policy experts, lawyers, and computer programmers who examine data from a variety of sources to expose threats to your health and the environment, and to find solutions.

WorldWatch Institute
www.worldwatch.org

> WorldWatch is an independent research group working for an environmentally sustainable and socially just society. An

excellent book published by WorldWatch Institute is Brian Halweil's *Eat Here: Reclaiming Homegrown Pleasures in a Global Supermarket*, 2004.

Global Resource Action Center for the Environment (GRACE)
www.gracelinks.org / www.factoryfarm.org

The GRACE Factory Farm Project (GFFP) works to create a sustainable food production system that is healthful and humane, economically viable, and environmentally sound.

Food and Water Watch (FWW)
www.foodandwaterwatch.org

FWW works on many food and water safety issues, including mad cow disease, genetic engineering, factory farming, rBGH, and irradiation.

Sierra Club
www.sierraclub.org/factoryfarms/resources

The Sierra Club is an environmental group working to promote and protect the earth's ecosystems and resources.

Animal Welfare

Humane Society of the united states (HSUS)
www.hsus.org/farm_animals/factory_farms

HSUS has worked since 1954 to promote the protection of all animals.

Humane Farming Association (HFA)
www.hfa.org/factory/index.html

HFA is an animal protection organization that campaigns against factory farming and slaughterhouse abuses. HFA is also home to the world's largest farm animal refuge.

Compassionate Consumers
www.compassionateconsumers.org

Compassionate Consumers was founded in 2003 by people concerned about animal welfare in the food industry. They are working to ensure that consumers can find out truthful information about how their food is produced.

NOTES

1. Tiaji Salaam-Blyther, "US and International Responses to the Global Spread of Avian Flu: Issues for Congress," CRS Report for Congress, May 1, 2006, www.fas.org/sgp/crs/misc/RL33219.pdf.

2. "Infectious Disease Society of America Avian Influenza (Bird Flu): Agricultural and Wildlife Considerations," May 12, 2006, www.cidrap.umn.edu/idsa/influenza/avianflu/biofacts/avflu.html.

3. "Fowl Play: The Poultry Industry's Central Role in the Bird Flu Crisis," GRAIN, February 2006, grain.org/briefings/?id=194.

4. "Avian influenza ('Bird Flu')—Fact Sheet," World Health Organization, February 2006, www.who.int/mediacentre/factsheets/avian_influenza/en/.

5. "Frequently Asked Questions About Bird Flu," Department of Health, Republic of the Philippines, www.doh.gov.ph/bird_flu.htm.

6. Drs. Tony Caver, Boyd Parr, Julie Helm, and Pam Parnell, "One Clemson Approach to Avian Influenza," Clemson University Livestock Poultry Health Division, May 20, 2006, www.clemson.edu/LPH/AIOneClemson52006.pdf.

7. "Case of Human Conjunctivitis Due to Low Pathogenicity H7N3 Avian Influenza in UK," European Center for Disease Prevention and Control, May 2, 2006, www.ecdc.eu.int/press/press_releases/PDF/060502.press_release.pdf.

8. A. J. Hostetler and Calvin Trice, "Va. Worker May Have Caught Avian Flu," *Times Dispatch*, February 28, 2004, www.timesdispatch.com/servlet/Satellite?pagename=RTD%2FMGArticle %2FRTD_BasicArticle&c=MGArticle&cid=1031773945646&path=%21news&s=1045855934842.

9. "Avian Influenza Infection in Humans," Centers for Disease Control, www.cdc.gov/flu/avian/gen-info/avian-flu-humans.htm.

10. "Avian Influenza (Bird Flu): Agricultural and Wildlife Considerations," Center for Infectious Disease Research & Policy, University of Minnesota. Last updated July 19, 2006. Accessed July 19, 2006, http://www.cidrap.umn.edu/cidrap/content/influenza/avianflu/biofacts/avflu.htm.

11. R. A. M. Fouchier, P. M. Schneeberger, F. W. Rozendaal et al., "Avian Influenza: A Virus (H7N7) Associated with Human Conjunctivitis and a Fatal Case of Acute Respiratory Distress Syndrome," *Proc Natl Acad Sci* 101, no. 5 (February 3, 2004): 1356–61 [Full text].

12. A. Stegeman, A. Bouma, A. R. W. Elbers et al., "Avian Influenza: A Virus (H7N7) Epidemic in The Netherlands in 2003: Course of the Epidemic and Effectiveness of Control Measures," *Journal of Infectious Diseases* 190 (December 15, 2004): 2088–95 [Abstract].

13. "Avian Influenza (Bird Flu): Agricultural and Wildlife Considerations," Center

for Infectious Disease Research & Policy, University of Minnesota. Last updated July 19, 2006. Accessed July 19, 2006, http://www.cidrap.umn.edu/cidrap/content/influenza/avianflu/biofacts/avflu.htm.

14. "Avian Influenza ('Bird Flu')—Fact Sheet," World Health Organization, February 2006, www.who.int/mediacentre/factsheets/avian_influenza/en/.

15. "A Closer Look at Bird Flu's Victim's," *Wall Street Journal Online*, July 19, 2006, daily updates, http://online.wsj.com/public/resources/documents/retro06 avfludeaths-date_desc.html?mod=blogs.

16. M. Alexander Otto, "Bird Flu Threat Not So Grave, CDC Chief Says," *News Tribune*, April 15, 2006, www.thenewstribune.com/health/story/5663764p-5080102c.html.

17. Ibid.

18. Ibid.

19. Ibid.

20. Ibid.

21. "Penn State Avian Influenza Experts Address Current Poultry and Human Health Issues Workshop," April 18, 2006, Farm Show Complex, Harrisburg, PA, www.cas.psu.edu/docs/biosecurity/avianfluvideos.html.

22. Rhiannon Coppin, "Foul Forecast," *The Vancouver Courier.com*, September 22, 2005, www.vancourier.com/issues05/093205/news/093205nn1.html.

23. Ibid.

24. Ibid.

25. Dr. Shiv Chopra, personal communication with author.

26. "Paranoia, Bird Flu and the World Health Org," *Maclean's*, May 22, 2006.

27. Donald G. McNeil Jr., "Avian Flu Wanes in Asia Nations It First Hit Hard," *New York Times*, May 14, 2006, www.nytimes.com/2006/05/14/world/asia/14flu.html?pagewanted=1&_r=2&th& emc=th.

28. Ibid.

29. Ibid.

30. Ibid.

31. Krishna Ramanujan, "Migratory Birds Are Unlikely to Infect Humans or Poultry in U.S. with Deadly Avian Flu, Say Cornell Bird Experts," April 26, 2006, http://www.news.cornell.edu/stories/April06/H5N1migration.ksr.html.

32. Anita Manning, "Bird Flu Is Taking a Bit of a Breather," *USA Today*, May 14, 2006, www.usatoday.com/news/health/2006-05-14-birdflu-spread_x.htm.

33. Ibid.

34. Joyce Howard Price, "Bird Flu Too Deep in Human Lungs to Spread Easily," *Washington Times*, March 23, 2006, www.washtimes.com/national/20060322-111957-5097r.htm.

35. Jia-Rui Chong, "Bird Flu Seems to Have Taken Deadly New Step in Indonesia," May 25, 2006, *Los Angeles Times*, www.latimes.com/news/science/la-sci-bird flu25may25,1,3060809.story?ctrack=1&cset=true.

36. Judith Graham, "Outbreak Has Bird-Flu Experts Stumped," *Chicago Tribune*, May 24, 2006, www.chicagotribune.com/news/custom/newsroom/chi-060524 bird-flu,1,2751614.story?coll=chi-news-hed&ctrack=1&cset=true.

37. "Human Spread No. 1 Suspect in Bird Flu Cluster," Associate Press, May 24, 2006, www.msnbc.msn.com/id/12939359/.

38. Ibid.

39. Elisabeth Rosenthal, "Human-to-Human Infection by Bird Flu Is Confirmed," *New York Times*, June 24, 2006, http://www.nytimes.com/2006/06/24/health/ 24flu.html?ei=5090&en=c1fc5b6aff481399&ex=1308801600&partner=rssuser land&emc=rss&pagewanted=print>confirmed.

40. Fred Francis, "Bird Flu Clusters Befuddle Doctors and Villagers," May 24, 2006, NBC News, www.msnbc.msn.com/id/12953295/.

41. "Cumulative Number of Confirmed Human Cases of Avian Influenza A/(H5N1) Reported to WHO," July 14, 2006, http://www.who.int/csr/ disease/avian_influenza/country/cases_table_2006_07_14/en/index.html.

42. "Audubon Society Avian Influenza Information," March 8, 2006, www.audubon.org/bird/avianflu/avianflu.htm.

43. "Clinical Description and Diagnosis, Hospitalizations and Deaths from Influenza," Centers for Disease Control, www.cdc.gov/flu/professionals/diagnosis/.

44. "Key Facts About Influenza and the Influenza Vaccine," Centers for Disease Control, www.cdc.gov/flu/keyfacts.htm.

45. Peter Doshi, "Are US Flu Death Figures More PR Than Science?" BMJ 331 (December 10, 2005): 1412, www.torstenengelbrecht.com/artikel_wissens chaft/BMJ_CDC_RKI_figures_Jan2005.pdf.

46. Glen Nowak, PhD, "Planning for the 2004–2005 Influenza Vaccine Season: A Communication Situation Analysis," www.ama-assn.org/ama1/pub/upload/mm/36/2004_flu_nowak.pdf.

47. Ibid.

48. "National Vital Statistics Reports," Centers for Disease Control, October 9, 2001, www.cdc.gov/nchs/data/nvsr/nvsr49/nvsr49_12.pdf.

49. "U.S. Centers for Disease Control Chronic Disease Overview," www.cdc.gov/nccdphp/overview.htm#2.

50. Ibid.

51. "Conditions by Deaths," CureResarch.com, 2005, www.cureresearch.com/lists/deaths.htm.

52. "Cholera," World Health Organization, Initiative for Vaccine Research (IVR), 2006, www.who.int/vaccine_research/diseases/diarrhoeal/en/index3.html.

53. "Infectious Diseases," Global Health Council, www.globalhealth.org/view_top.php3?id=228.

54. Dr. William Legett Aldis, "Celebrating Water for Life," World Water Day, March 22, 2005, www.unescap.org/esd/water/events/wwd/2005/documents/WHO.doc.

55. Ibid.

56. "The London Plague of 1665," Britain Express, www.britainexpress.com/History/plague.htm.

57. Gina Kolata, *Flu: The Story of the Great Influenza Pandemic* (New York: Touchstone, 1999).

58. David M. Rorvick, "Of Ida Honorof, Defoliants, Deformed Babies, Legal Manslaughter, The EPA, Cancer and You," www.aliciapatterson.org/APF001976/Rorvik/Rorvik03/Rorvik03.html.

59. "Romania Maintains Bird Flu Quarantines," National Public Radio, May 24, 2006, www.npr.org/templates/story/story.php?storyId=5428491.

60. "Fowl Play: The Poultry Industry's Central Role in the Bird Flu Crisis," GRAIN, February, 2006, www.grain.org/briefings/?id=194.

61. "Grippe Aviaire-M. le Minister, la Paysannerie Ne Veut Pas de Votre Argent! Levez le Confinement," press release, *Union Paysanne*, May 6, 2006, www.unionpaysanne.com.

62. "Bird Flu History," The Bird Flu, www.bird-flu-clues.com/bird_flu_history.html.

63. "Avian Influenza Infection in Humans," Centers for Disease Control, April 24, 2006, www.cdc.gov/flu/avian/gen-info/avian-flu-humans.htm.

64. "H5N1 Avian Influenza: Timeline," World Health Organization, May 8, 2006, www.who.int/csr/disease/avian_influenza/timeline.pdf.

CHAPTER TWO

1. Danny Schechter, "The Media Shift from Them to Us," Common Dreams, May 8, 2006, www.commondreams.org/views06/0508-21.htm.

2. Nelson Thall, personal communication with author.

3. George Orwell, *1984* (London: Secker and Warburg, 1949).

4. John B. Horrigan, "Home Broadband Adoption 2006," Pew Internet & American Life Project, May 28, 2006, http://www.pewinternet.org/pdfs/PIP_Broadband_trends2006.pdf.

5. Pew Internet & American Life Project Surveys, March 2000–April 2006, http://www.pewinternet.org/trends/Internet_Adoption_4.26.06.pdf.

6. John B. Horrigan, "Home Broadband Adoption 2006," Pew Internet & American Life Project, May 28, 2006, www.pewinternet.org/pdfs/PIP_Broadband_trends2006.pdf.

7. Ibid.

8. John B. Horrigan, "For Many Home Broadband Users, the Internet Is a Primary News Source," Pew Internet & American Life Project, March 22, 2006, http://www.pewinternet.org/pdfs/PIP_News.and.Broadband.pdf.

9. Nicolas Johnson, "Take This Media . . . Please!" *Nation*, January 7, 2002.

10. Dr. Tim O'Shea, *The Doors of Perception: Why Americans Will Believe Almost Anything*, August 15, 2001, www.mercola.com/2001/aug/15/perception.htm.

11. "U.S. Issues $1 Billion in Flu Vaccine Contracts," Reuters, May 5, 2006, www.theepochtimes.com/news/6-5-5/41200.html.

12. Hal Boedecker, *Orlando Sentinel*, blogs.orlandosentinel.com/entertainment_tv_tvblog/nbc/index.html.

13. *Washington Post*-ABC News Poll, www.washingtonpost.com/wp-srv/politics/includes/postpoll_iraqwar_030606.htm.

14. Paul Blaum and Vicki Fong, *Pharmaceutical Ads Mix Information with Emotion*, Penn State University, June 2, 2000, http://www.psu.edu/ur/2000/drugads.html.

15. Barbara Mintzes, "Direct-to-Consumer Advertising of Prescription Drugs— Whatever the Problem, You Can Always Pop a Pill," CEWH Research Bulletin, Spring 2003, volume 3, number 2, http://www.cewh-cesf.ca/bulletin/v3n2/page5.html.

16a. "How Journalists See Journalists in 2004," Pew Research Center for the People and the Press, June 2004, http://people-press.org/reports/pdf/214.pdf.

16b. "Public More Critical of Press but Goodwill Persists," Pew Research Center for the People and the Press, June 2005, http://people-press.org/reports/pdf/248.pdf; www.stateofthenewsmedia.org/2006/narrative_networktv_publicattitudes.asp?cat=7&media=5.

16c. Ibid,

17. Leonard Downie Jr. and Robert Kaiser, *The News About the News: American Journalism in Peril*, Knopf, 2002.

18. Phil Donahue, interview with Independent World Television, 2005.

19. Leslie Cauley, "NSA Has Massive Database of Amercan's Phone Calls," *USA Today*, May 11, 2006, www.usatoday.com/news/washington/2006-05-10-nsa_x.htm.

20. Richard Morin, "Poll—Most Americans Support NSA's Efforts," *Washington Post*, May 12, 2006, www.washingtonpost.com/wp-dyn/content/article/2006/05/12/AR2006051200375_pf.html.

21. Steven Reinberg, "One-Third of U.S. Adults Diabetic or Pre-Diabetic," Yahoo! News, May 26, 2006, news.yahoo.com/s/hsn/20060526/hl_hsn/onethirdofusadultsdiabeticorprediabetic.

22. Catherine C. Cowie, PhD, Keith F. Rust, PhD, Danita D. Byrd-Holt, BBA, Mark S. Eberhardt, PhD, Katherine M. Flegal, PhD, Michael M. Engelgau, MD, Sharon H. Saydah, PhD, Desmond E. Williams, MD, Linda S. Geiss, MS, and Edward W. Gregg, PhD, "Prevalence of Diabetes and Impaired Fasting Glucose in Adults in the U.S. Population," *Diabetes Care* 29 (June 2006): 1263–68.

23. D. A. Bennett, MD, J. A. Schneider, MD, J. L. Bienias, ScD, D. A. Evans, MD, and R. S. Wilson, PhD, "Mild Cognitive Impairment Is Related to Alzheimer Disease Pathology and Cerebral Infarctions," *Neurology* 64 (March 8, 2005): 834–41.

24. A. Jemal, T. Murray, E. Ward, A. Samuels, R. C. Tiwari, A. Ghafoor, E. J. Feuer, and M. J. Thun, "Cancer Statistics 2005," *CA Cancer J Cli*, 55, no. 1 (January/February 2005): 10–30.

25. "Cancer Now the Top Killer of Americans," *USA Today*, January 19, 2005, www.usatoday.com/news/health/2005-01-19-cancer-deaths_x.htm.

26. "Rank Order—Life Expectancy at Birth," CIA World Factbook, 2006, www.cia.gov/cia/publications/factbook/rankorder/2102rank.html.

27. "The Medical Mafia—Pam Killeen Interviews Ghislaine Lactôt," *Crusador* 28 (December/January 2005/6).

28. "Fluoride Industry Busted—Pam Killeen Interviews Dr. Paul Connett," *Crusador* 27. (October/November 2005).

29. Jennifer Washburn, *University Inc.: The Corporate Corruption of Higher Education* (Cambridge: Perseus Books Group, 2005).

30. "Fluoride Industry Busted—Pam Killeen Interviews Dr. Paul Connett," *Crusador* 27 (October/November 2005).

31. Jeffrey H. Birnbaum, "The Road to Riches Is Called K Street," *Washington Post*, June 22, 2005, www.washingtonpost.com/wp-dyn/content/article/2005/06/21/AR2005062101632.html.

32. "Congressional Revolving Doors: The Journey from Congress to K Street," Public Citizen Congress Watch, July, 2005, http://www.lobbyinginfo.org/documents/RevolveDoor.pdf.

33. Anna Lappé and Bryant Terry, *Grub: Ideas for an Urban Kitchen* (New York: Penguin Group, 2006), 45.

34. Ibid.

35. Rep. Henry A. Waxman, "Politics and Science in the Bush Administration," United States House Representatives Committee on Government Reform—Minority Staff Special Investigations Division, August 2003, www.house.gov/reform/min/politicsandscience/pdfs/pdf_politics_and_science_rep.pdf.

36. Luise Light, personal communication with author.

37. "Foodborne Illness," Centers for Disease Control and Prevention, www.cdc.gov/ncidod/dbmd/diseaseinfo/foodborneinfections_t.htm.

38. Ibid.

39. Luise Light, M.S., Ed.D. personal communication with author.

40. Edward L. Bernays, *Propaganda* (Brooklyn: Ig Publishing, 2004).

41. Anna Lappé and Bryant Terry, *Grub: Ideas for an Urban Kitchen* (New York: Penguin Group, 2006), 44.

42. Ibid.

43. National Health Information Center, U.S. Department of Health and Human Services; Health Information Resource Database—Calorie Control Council, www.health.gov/nhic/Scripts/Entry.cfm?HRCode=HR1137.

44. Anna Lappé and Bryant Terry, *Grub: Ideas for an Urban Kitchen* (Penguin Group, 2006), 44.

45. Ibid.

46. Ibid., 43.

47. Center for Global Food Issues, Source Watch, www.sourcewatch.org/index. php?title=Center_for_Global_Food_Issues.

48. Ibid.

49. Anna Lappé and Bryant Terry, *Grub: Ideas for an Urban Kitchen* (New York: Penguin Group, 2006), 75.

50. Center for Consumer Freedom, Source Watch, www.sourcewatch.org/index.php? title=Center_for_Consumer_Freedom.

51. Ibid.

52. "New FDA Report Threatens Consumer Choices: Big Government Wants Restaurants to Force Their Customers to Eat Brussels Sprouts," June 2, 2006, www.consumerfreedom.com/pressRelease_detail.cfm/release/157.

53. "Needless Fish Warnings Not Good 'Science,' Not 'In the Public Interest,'" The Center for Consumer Freedom, July 6, 2006, http://www.consumerfreedom.com/ pressRelease_detail.cfm/release/162.

54. "A Band-Aid for Obesity," The Center for Consumer Freedom, April 7, 2006, http://www.consumerfreedom.com/news_detail.cfm/headline/3007.

55. Sheldon Rampton and John Stauber, *Trust Us—We're Experts* (New York: Tarcher/ Penguin, 2001), 22.

56. Ibid.

57. "Fake TV News: News Release, Investigation Catches 77 Local TV Stations Presenting Corporate PR as Real News," April 6, 2006, www.prwatch.org/fakenews/ release.

58. Ibid.

59. Ibid.

60. Ibid.

61. Diane Farsetta and Daniel Price, "Fake TV News: Widespread and Undisclosed," Center for Media and Democracy, April 6, 2006,www.prwatch.org/ map/TV_Stations.

62. David Miller, "Democracy: Corporate Spin's Part in Its Downfall," May 19, 2006, www.spinwatch.org.

63. "Public More Critical of Press, but Goodwill Persists," Pew Research Center for People and the Press, June 26, 2005, http://people-press.org/reports/pdf/248. pdf.

Chapter Three

1. "Jerry Kay Interview with Michael Pollan, Author of The Omnivore's Dilemma," Beyond Organic, April 19, 2006, www.beyondorganic.com/shows/ beyondorganic041906.mp3.

2. Mary Zanoni, PhD, JD, "NAIS: A New Threat to Rural Freedom," *Hobby Farms.com Magazine*, January/February 2006; article originally published in *Countryside & Small Stock Journal*, January/February 2006.

3. Ibid.

4. USDA Draft Strategic Plan, 4, published April 25, 2005.
5. Mary Zanoni, PhD, JD, "The 'National Animal Identification System': A New Threat to Rural Freedom," *Countryside & Small Stock Journal*, January/February 2006.
6. "Who Will Feed the Inmates?" Rural Advancement Foundation International, August 31 2000, www.etcgroup.org/documents/geno_prisoners.pdf.
7. "A History of American Agriculture 1776-1990," inventors.about.com/library/inventors/blfarm4.htm.
8. U.S. Department of Labor, Bureau of Labor Statistics, Farmers, Ranchers, and Agricultural Managers, www.bls.gov/oco/ocos176.htm.
9. Dan Morgan, Gilbert M. Gaul, and Sarah Cohen, "Farm Program Pays $1.3 Billion to People Who Don't Farm," *Washington Post*, July 2, 2006,www. washingtonpost.com/wp-dyn/content/article/2006/07/01/AR2006070100962. html?sub=AR.
10. Lynn R. Miller, "USDA Poised to Push Us Off Our Farms with NAIS," *Small Farmers Journal*, Winter 2006, http://www.smallfarmersjournal.com/images/NAIS_editorial_Lynn_Miller.pdf.
11. Ibid.
12. Judith McGeary, "Follow the Money," Farm and Ranch Freedom Alliance, http://www.farmandranchfreedom.org/money.html.
13. Judith McGeary personal communication with author.
14. Judith McGeary, JD, "Analysis of the NAIS and Proposed Texas Regulations," March 20, 2006, www.farmandranchfreedom.org/analysis_nais.html.
15. "Animal ID," Food and Water Watch Alert, May 19, 2006,www.foodandwaterwatch. org/food/factoryfarms/animal-i-d.
16. Amanda Griscom Little, "Old Big Brother Had a Farm," Grist, March 10, 2006, www.grist.org/news/muck/2006/03/10/griscom-little/.
17. Ibid.
18. Jedd Kettler, "Big Brother on the Animal Farm? Animal ID System Raises Orwellian Concerns for Some," *Franklin County Farmer* 14 (Spring 2006), www. thecountycourier.com/index.php?option=content&task=view&id=2859&Itemid.
19. "Homeland Security: Much Is Being Done to Protect Agriculture from a Terrorist Attack, but Important Challenges Remain," United States Government Accountability Office, GAO-05-214, March 2005.
20. Jedd Kettler; "Big Brother on the Animal Farm? Animal ID System Raises Orwellian Concerns for Some," *Franklin County Farmer* 14 (Spring 2006), www. thecountycourier.com/index.php?option=content&task=view&id=2859&Itemid.
21. Ibid.
22. "Concentrated Animal Feeding Operations (CAFOs), About CAFOs," National Center for Environmental Health, CDC, www.cdc.gov/CAFOs/about.htm.
23. Danielle Nierenberg (Project Director), "State of the World 2006," WorldWatch Institute, 2006.

24. Karen Davis, PhD, "The Ethics of Genetic Engineering and the Futuristic Fate of Domestic Fowl," The Ethics of Genetic Engineering and Animal Patents Conference, October 12, 1996, www.upc-online.org/genetic.html.

25. "Facts About Our Food, Broiler Chickens," Canadian Coalition for Farm Animals, www.humanefood.ca/docs/FactSheets/Broiler2004.pdf.

26. "Factory Farming: Concentrated Animal Feeding Operations and the Poultry Industry," The Food Museum: CAFO Issue, www.foodmuseum.com/issuecafo.html.

27. Ibid.

28. David Wallinga, MD, "Playing Chicken: Avoiding Arsenic in Your Meat," Institute for Agricultural and Trade Policy, April 2006, www.environmentalobservatory.org/library.cfm?refid=80529.

29. Ibid.

30. Betty S. King, Janet Tietyen, and Steven S Vicker, "Food and Agriculture: Consumer Trends and Opportunities," University of Kentucky, www.ca.uky.edu/agc/pubs/ip/ip58f/IP58F.pdf.

31. David Wallinga, MD, "Playing Chicken: Avoiding Arsenic in Your Meat," Institute for Agricultural and Trade Policy, April 2006, www.environmentalobservatory.org/library.cfm?refid=80529.

32. Danielle Nierenberg, "Happier Meals: Rethinking the Global Meat Industry," WorldWatch, September 2005.

33. Ibid.

34. "Fowl Play: The Poultry Industry's Central Role in the Bird Flu Crisis," GRAIN, February 2006, www.grain.org/briefings/?id=194.

35. Dr. Shiv Chopra personal communication with author.

36. "WHO: Bird Droppings Prime Origin of Bird Flu," China Daily, January 17, 2004, www.china.org.cn/english/scitech/84972.htm.

37. F. William Engdahl, "Bird Flu and Chicken Factory Farms: Profit Bonanza for U.S. Agribusiness," Global Research.ca, November 27, 2005, www.globalresearch.ca/index.php?context=viewArticle&code=ENG20051127&articleId=1333.

38. Wendy Orent, "The Price of Cheap Chicken Is Bird Flu," op-ed, LA Times.com, March 12, 2006, www.latimes.com/news/opinion/sunday/commentary/la-op-orent12mar12,0,6380375.story?coll=la-sunday-commentary.

39. Mae-Wan Ho, "Fowl Play in Bird Flu," Institute of Science in Society, May 5, 2006. http://www.i-sis.org.uk/Fowl-Play-in-Bird-Flu.php.

40. "Fowl Play: The Poultry Industry's Central Role in Bird Flu Crisis," GRAIN, February 2006, http://www.grain.org/briefings/?id=194.

41. Ibid.

42. Dr. Paul Aho, "The Outlook for Asian Feed Demand," USDA Outlook Forum, February 17, 2006, www.usda.gov/oce/forum/2006%20Speeches/PDF%20PPT/Aho.pdf.

43. Ibid.

44. "Avian Flu: No Need to Kill Wild Birds," FAO Newsroom, July 16, 2004, http://www.fao.org/newsroom/en/news/2004/48287/index.html.

45. Michael Satchell and Stephen J. Hedges. "The Next Bad Beef Scandal?" *US News and World Report*, September 1, 1997, www.organicconsumers.org/shit.html.

46. "WHO: Bird Droppings Prime Origin of Bird Flu," *China Daily*, January 17, 2004, www.china.org.cn/english/scitech/84972.htm.

47. David Wallinga, MD, "Playing Chicken: Avoiding Arsenic in Your Meat," Institute for Agricultural and Trade Policy, April 2006, www.environmentalobservatory. org/library.cfm?refid=80529.

48. Ibid.

49. Suzi Parker, "Finger-Lickin' Bad: How Poultry Producers Are Ravaging the Rural South," *Grist Magazine*, February 21, 2006, www.grist.org/news/maindish/ 2006/02/21/parker/.

50. Ibid.

51. Ibid.

52. Suzi Parker. "Finger-Lickin' Bad: How Poultry Producers Are Ravaging the Rural South," *Grist Magazine*, Febraru 21, 2006, www.grist.org/news/maindish/ 2006/02/21/parker/.

53. Ron Wood, "Judge Considers Motion to Dismiss Lawsuit,: The Morning News, June 21, 2006.

54. Professor C. J. Feare, "Fish Farming and the Risk of Spread of Avian Influenza," Bird Life International, March 2006, www.birdlife.org/action/science/species/avian_flu/pdfs/fish_farming_review.pdf.

55. Michael McCarthy, "Bird Flu Could Be Linked to Fish Farming," *New Zealand Herald*, December 28, 2005, www.nzherald.co.nz/section/story.cfm?c_id=5& objectid=10361729.

56. "UN Vet Dismisses Fish Farming as Bird Flu Risk," Reuters, December 29, 2005, www.planetark.com/dailynewsstory.cfm/newsid/34241/story.htm.

57. Christoph Scholtissek and Ernest Naylor, "Fish Farming and Influenza Pandemics," *Nature* 331, no. 215 (January 21, 1988).

58. Dr. Martin Williams, "Farm Fish Fed Dead Chickens a Risk for H5N1 Influenza in Indonesia?" April 10, 2006, www.drmartinwilliams.com/conservation/cat fish-farm.html.

59. Christoph Scholtissek and Ernest Naylor, "Fish Farming and Influenza Pandemics," *Nature* 331, no. 215 (January 21, 1988).

60. Professor C. J Feare, "Fish Farming and the Risk of Spread of Avian Influenza," Bird Life International, March 2006, http://www.birdlife.org/action/science/ species/avian_flu/pdfs/fish_farming_review.pdf.

61. M. Nathaniel Mead, "Arsenic: A Global Poison," *Environmental Health Perspectives* 113, no. 6 (June 2005).

62. Ibid.

63. Ibid.

64. David Wallinga, MD, "Playing Chicken: Avoiding Arsenic in Your Meat," Institute for Agricultural and Trade Policy, April 2006, www.environmentalobservatory. org/library.cfm?refid=80529.

65. Maureen Rouhi, "Arsenic in Rice," *Chemical & Engineering News* 83, no. 32 (August 3, 2005): 14. (RE: Environ. Sci. Technol. 2005, 39, 5531)

66. David Wallinga, MD, "Playing Chicken: Avoiding Arsenic in Your Meat," Institute for Agricultural and Trade Policy, April 2006, www.environmentalobservatory. org/library.cfm?refid=80529.

67. Ibid.

68. Ibid.

69. *Wegmans Cruelty*, A film by Compassionate Consumers, 2005, www.wegmans cruelty.com/content/blogcategory/20/36/.

70. Ibid.

71. Patrick Condon, "Better Business Bureau Nixes Egg Ads," Associated Press, May 11, 2004, http://www.thelocalbbb.org/alerts/alerts.html?newsid=381& newstype=1.

72. "Business Group Shells Egg Industry Ads," MSNBC, May 11, 2004. http:// www.msnbc.msn.com/id/4951194/.

73. Wegmans Cruelty, A film by Compassionate Consumers, 2005, www.wegmans cruelty.com/content/blogcategory/20/36/.

74. Patrick Condon, "Better Business Bureau Nixes Egg Ads," Associated Press, May 11, 2004, http://www.thelocalbbb.org/alerts/alerts.html?newsid=381& newstype=1.

75. "Business Group Shells Egg Industry Ads," MSNBC, May 11, 2004, http:// www.msnbc.msn.com/id/4951194/.

76. Krestia Degeorge, "Jailing a Cage-Free Activist," *Rochester City News*, May 24, 2006, www.rochester-citynews.com/gyrobase/Content?oid=oid%3A4438.

77. Center for Media and Democracy, Source Watch, Center for Consumer Freedom, http://www.sourcewatch.org/index.php?title=Center_for_Consumer_Freedom.

78. "Putting People Over Poultry," The Center for Consumer Freedom, May 26, 2006, www.consumerfreedom.com/news_detail.cfm/headline/3041.

79. M. H. Birley and K. Lock, "The Health Impacts of Peri-urban Natural Resource Development, International Center for Health Impact Assessment," Liverpool, England, 1999, 85, www.ihia.org.uk/document/periurbanhia.pdf.

80. D. M. Mannino, J. E. Parker, and M. C. Townsend, "Dairy Farming Production in the US and Death with Farmer's Lung from 1976–1986: An Ecological Study," *American Review of RespiratoryDisease* 141 (1990): A588.

81. Luladey B. Tadesse, "Poultry Workers Carrying Resistant Bacteria, Study Finds, Researchers Target Employees, Growers, on Delmarva," May 12, 2006, www. delawareonline.com/apps/pbcs.dll/article?AID=/20060512/NEWS/605120340/1006.

82. Ibid.

83. Suzi Parker, "Finger-Lickin' Bad: How Poultry Producers Are Ravaging the Rural

South," *Grist Magazine*, Febraruy 21, 2006, www.grist.org/news/maindish/2006/02/21/parker/.

84. Ibid.

85. Corporate Power, www.yorku.ca/cculture/new%20website/C-Culture/website/corporate.htm.

86. Doug McInnis, "Super Chicken," *Beef Magazine,* February 1, 2000, beef-mag.com/mag/beef_super_chicken/index.html.

87. Charles Margulis personal communication with author.

88. B. Olsen, V. J. Munster, A. Wallensten, J. Waldenstrom, A. D. M. E, Osterhaus, and A. M. Fouchier, "Global Patterns of Influenza A Virus in Wild Birds," *Science* 312 (2006): 384–88.

CHAPTER FOUR

1. "Testing Birds for Bird Flu Begins in Alaska," Associated Press, May 19, 2006, www.cnn.com/2006/HEALTH/05/19/birdflu.testing.ap/index.html.

2. Anita Manning, "Bird Flu Is Taking a Bit of a Breather," *USA Today*, May 14, 2006, www.usatoday.com/news/health/2006-05-14-birdflu-spread_x.htm.

3. "Fowl Play: The Poultry Industry's Central Role in the Bird Flu Crisis," GRAIN, February 2006, http://www.grain.org/briefings/?id=194.

4. "Avian Flu: No Need to Kill Wild Birds," FAO Newsroom, July 16, 2004, www.fao.org/newsroom/en/news/2004/48287/index.html.

5. "Wild Bird Flu Blame 'Too Hasty,'" BBC News, January 24, 2006, http://news.bbc.co.uk/2/hi/europe/4642008.stm.

6. "Fowl Play: The Poultry Industry's Central Role in Bird Flu Crisis, GRAIN, February 2006, http://www.grain.org/briefings/?id=194.

7. "Birdwatch Ireland Update on Avian Flu Influenza—Bird Flu," www.birdwatchireland.ie/bwi/pages092003/news/newsfaq_avianflu.html.

8. Bill Engdahl, "Bird Flu and Chicken Factory Farms: Profit Bonanza for U.S. Agribusiness," Global Research, November 27, 2005,www.globalresearch.ca/index.php?context=viewArticle&code=ENG20051127&articleId=1333.

9. Isabelle Delforge, "The Flu That Made Agribusiness Stronger," Focus on the Global South, July 5, 2004 [article first appeared in *Bangkok Post*], www.focusweb.org/content/view/363/28/ .

10. Ibid.

11. Richard Hobday, *The Healing Sun Sunlight and Health in the 21st Century* (London: Finhorn Press, 1999).

12. P. T. Liu, S. Stenge et al., "Toll-Like Receptor Triggering of a Vitamin D-Mediated Human Antimicrobial Response," *Science* 311, no. 5768 (March 24, 2006): 1770–73 [Epub February 23, 2006].

13. Joel Salatin, personal communication with author.

14. Stella Purdy, personal communication with author.

15. Ibid.

16. "The Top-Down Global Response to Bird Flu," GRAIN, April 2006, grain.org/articles/?id=12#sdfootnote1sym.

17. "World Health Organization, Avian Influenza ('Bird Flu') Fact Sheet," 2006, www.who.int/mediacentre/factsheets/avian_influenza/en/index.html#birds.

18. "The Top-Down Global Response to Bird Flu," GRAIN, April 2006, grain.org/articles/?id=12#sdfootnote1sym.

19. "Fowl Play: The Poultry Industry's Central Role in Bird Flu Crisis," GRAIN, February 2006, http://www.grain.org/briefings/?id=194.

20. Ibid.

21. Dr. Eva Wallner-Pendleton, DVM, MS, DACPV, "Protecting Small Flocks from Avian Influenza," Workshop, April 18, 2006, Harrisburg, PA, www.cas.psu.edu/docs/biosecurity/avianfluvideos.html.

22. Dr. Paul Aho, "The Outlook for Asian Feed Demand," USDA Agricultural Outlook Forum, February 17, 2006, Washington DC, www.usda.gov/oce/forum/2006%20Speeches/PDF%20PPT/Aho.pdf.

23. Dr. Paul Aho, "The Outlook for Asian Feed Demand," USDA Agricultural Outlook Forum, February 17, 2006, Washington DC, http://www.usda.gov/oce/forum/2006%20Speeches/PDF%20PPT/Aho.pdf.

24. Dr. Mae-Wan Ho, "Fowl Play in Bird Flu," Institute of Science in Society, May 5, 2006, www.i-sis.org.uk/Fowl-Play-in-Bird-Flu.php.

25. T. Tiensin, P. Chaitaweesub, T. Songserm, A. Chaisingh, W. Hoonsuwan, C. Buranathai, T. Parakamawongsa, S. Premashthira, A. Amonsin, M. Gilber, M. Nielen, and A. Stegeman, "Highly Pathogenic Avian Influenza H5N1,Thailand, 2004," *Emerging Infectious Disease* 11 (2005): 1664-72.

26. Dr. Mae-Wan Ho, "Fowl Play in Bird Flu, Institute of Science in Society," May 5, 2006, www.i-sis.org.uk/Fowl-Play-in-Bird-Flu.php.

27. Joel Salatin, personal communication with author.

28. Ibid.

29. Ibid.

30. "Fact Sheet: Market Impact of Avian Flu in Asia," Food and Agriculture Organization, www.fao.org/ES/ESC/en/20953/21014/highlight_36567en.html.

31. Ibid.

32. Bill Engdahl, "Bird Flu and Chicken Factory Farms: Profit Bonanza for U.S. Agribusiness," Global Research, November 27, 2005, www.globalresearch.ca/index.php?context=viewArticle&code=ENG20051127&articleId=1333.

33. Wendy Orent, "The Price of Cheap Chicken Is Bird Flu," *LATimes.com*, March 12, 2006, www.latimes.com/news/opinion/sunday/commentary/la-op-orent12mar12,0,6380375.story?coll=la-sunday-commentary.

34. Isabelle Delforge, "The Flu That Made Agribusiness Stronger," Focus on the Global South, July 5, 2004, www.focusweb.org/content/view/363/28/.

35. Isabelle Delforge, "Thailand: The World's Kitchen," *Le Monde Diplomatique*, July 2004, mondediplo.com/2004/07/05thailand.

36. Ibid.

37. Shelley Page, "In the End, the 'Egg Police' Chickened Out," *Ottawa Citizen*, September 12, 2005, www.vivelecanada.ca/forum/viewtopic.php?forum=28&showtopic=13009.

38. Ibid.

39. Maureen Bostock, "Egg Grading Is Not a Health Necessity," letter to the editor, *Ottawa Citizen*, September 14, 2005, www.ruralcouncil.ca/egg-war-050912.htm.

40. Ibid.

41. Ibid.

42. Dr. Mae-Wan Ho, "What Can You Believe About the Bird Flu," Institute of Science in Society, May 18, 2006.

43. Ibid.

44. Congressman George Miller (D-California, 7th District), Committee on Education and the Workforce, Committee on Resources, "Bush Administration Spent over $1.6 Billion on Advertising and Public Relations Contracts Since 2003, GAO Finds," press release, February 13, 2006, www.house.gov/georgemiller/press/rel21306.html.

45. Florence Nightingale, *Notes on Nursing* (New York: D. Appleton and Company, 1860).

46. Charles Walters, personal communication with author.

47. "Corporate Power," www.yorku.ca/cculture/new%20website/C-Culture/website/corporate.htm.

48. Charles Walters, personal communication with author.

49. David Wallinga, "Playing Chicken: Avoiding Arsenic in Your Meat," Institute of Agriculture and Trade Policy, April 2006, http://www.environmentalobservatory.org/library.cfm?refid=80529.

50. "Why McDonald's Fries Taste So Good—01.01," *Atlantic Monthly* 287, no. 1 (January 2001): 50–56.

51. "Cage-free Hens Pushed to Rule Roost," *USA Today*, April 10, 2006, www.usatoday.com/news/health/2006-04-10-eggs-cage_x.htm.

CHAPTER FIVE

1. Aaron Smith, "U.S. Gears Up for Anthrax, Smallpox," CNN/Money, September 16 2005, money.cnn.com/2005/09/16/news/fortune500/stockpile/index.htm.

2. "Viragen Reports Achievement of Key Avian Transgenics Milestone," June 3, 2005, www.prnewswire.com/mnr/viragen/22034/.

3. Viragen, OVA™ System (Avian Transgenics), www.viragen.com/aviantransgenicbio.htm.

4. Ibid.

5. Ibid.

6. Mark Henderson, "Scientists Aim to Beat Flu with Genetically Modified

Chickens," *Times Online*, October 29, 2005, www.timesonline.co.uk/article/0,,25149-1847760,00.html.

7. Ibid.

8. United State Patent Office, www.ptos.org/pages.php?menuid=29.

9. Scott Killman, "U.S. Supreme Court Upholds the Right to Patent Plants," *Wall Street Journal*, December 12, 2001, http://www.biotech-info.net/upholds_right.html.

10. Ibid.

11. Jeffrey Smith, *Seeds of Deceptions: Exposing Industry and Government Lies About the Safety of the Genetically Engineered Foods You're Eating* (Fairfield: Yes! Books, 2003).

12. "Senate Backs $8 Billion for Bird-Flu Plan," Washington (UPI), October 27, 2005, www.terradaily.com/reports/Senate_Backs_$8_Billion_For_BirdFlu_Plan.html.

13. Richard Cowan, "Senate OK's $8 Billion to Fight Bird Flu," Reuters, October 27, 2005, mmrs.fema.gov/news/influenza/2005/oct/nflu2005-10-28a.aspx.

14. "Senate Backs $8 Billion for Bird-Flu Plan," Washington (UPI), October 27, 2005, www.terradaily.com/reports/Senate_Backs_$8_Billion_For_BirdFlu_Plan.html.

15. Todd Zwillich, "Senate Debates $8 Billion for Bird Flu Plan," WebMD Medical News, October 26, 2005, www.webmd.com/content/article/114/111236.htm.

16. "President's Letter for the National Strategy for Pandemic Influenza," November 1, 2005, WhiteHouse.Gov www.whitehouse.gov/homeland/nspi.pdf.

17. Sabin Russell, "Bush Urges $7.1 Billion Flu Fight Defense Against a Pandemic of Bird-Killing Strain," *San Francisco Chronicle*, November 2, 2005, www.sfgate.com/cgi-bin/article.cgi?f=/c/a/2005/11/02/MNG0DFHNR91.DTL.

18. Lawrence K. Altman. "Draft Report Outlines Plans for Pandemic," *New York Times*, May 3, 2006, www.nytimes.com/2006/05/03/washington/03flu.html?ex=1149220800&en=ed91a1fe16c27ddd&ei=5070.

19. "Bird Flu—the facts," *Londoner*, December 2005, www.london.gov.uk/londoner/05dec/p17a.jsp?nav=health.

20. "Tamiflu: Worth 'Considering,' Effective Measure," March 1, 2005, effectmeasure.blogspot.com/2005/03/tamiflu-worth-considering.html.

21. Dr. Mae-Wan Ho, "Where's the Bird Flu Pandemic?" Intitute of Science in Society, May 11, 2006.

22. "Virus Expert Questions Amount of Canada's Tamiflu Stockpiles," CBC, October 27, 2005, www.cbc.ca/story/science/national/2005/10/27/Tamiflu-051027.html.

23. "Rumsfeld's Growing Stake in Tamiflu," CNN, October 31, 2005, money.cnn.com/2005/10/31/news/newsmakers/fortune_rumsfeld/.

24. Bill Engdahl, "Is Avian Flu Another Pentagon Hoax?" Global Research, October 30 2005, www.globalresearch.ca/index.php?context=viewArticle&code=%20EN20051030&articleId=1169.

25. "Rumsfeld's Growing Stake in Tamiflu," CNN, October 31, 2005, money.cnn.com/2005/10/31/news/newsmakers/fortune_rumsfeld/.

26. Geoffrey Lean and Jonathan Owen, "Donald Rumsfeld Makes $5 Million Killing on Bird Flu Drug," Common Dreams.org, March 12, 2006. Original article from *Independent News*, UK, www.commondreams.org/headlines06/0312-06.htm.

27. T. Jefferson et al., "Antivirals for Influenza in Healthy Adults: Systematic Review," *Lancet* 367 (2006): 303-13.

28. "Health Canada Looking at Tamiflu Data After Reports of Deaths in Japan," Canadian Press, November 17, 2005, www.canada.com/health/story.html?id=d155eac6-df71-4639-a222-aee4d88f426c.

29. Anita Manning, "Roche Boosts Tamiflu Production," *USA Today*, March 16, 2006, www.usatoday.com/news/health/2006-03-16-tamiflu_x.htm.

30. Ibid.

31. "Frequently Asked Questions to Help You Feel Better," Tamiflu.com, www.tamiflu.com/faq_tamiflu.asp.

32. Dr. Shiv Chopra, personal communication with author.

33. Sherri Tenpenny, *Fowl: Bird Flu, It's Not What You Think* (Sevierville: Insight, 2006).

34. M. N. Matrosovich, T. Y. Matrosovich, T. Gray, N. A. Roberts, and H. D. Klenk, "Neuraminidase Is Important for the Initiation of Influenza Virus Infection in Human Airway Rpithelium," J Virol 78, no. 22 (November 2004): 12665-67.

35. I. V. Alymova, G. Taylor, and A. Portner, "Neuraminidase Inhibitors as Antiviral Agents," Curr Drug Targets Infect Disord 5, no. 4 (December 2005): 401-9.

36. Sherri Tenpenny, *Fowl: Bird Flu, It's Not What You Think* (Sevierville:Insight, 2006).

37. Ibid.

38. Menno D. de Jong MD, T. Tran, H. K. Truong et. al., "Oseltamivir Resistance During Treatment of Influenza A (H5N1) Infection," *New England Journal of Medicine* 353, no. 25 (December 2005): 2667-72.

39. Q. M. Le, M. Kiso, K. Someya et. al., "Avian Flu: Isolation of Drug-Resistant H5N1 Virus," *Nature* 437, no. 7062 (October 2005): 1108.

40. R. K. Gupta and J. S. Nguyen-Van-Tam, "Oseltamivir Resistance in Influenza A (H5N1) Infection," *New England Journal of Medicine* 354, no. 13 (March 30, 2006): 1423-24.

41. A. Moscona, "Oseltamivir Resistance—Disabling Our Influenza Defenses," *New England Journal of Medicine* 353, no. 25 (December 22, 2005): 2633-36.

42. Ibid.

43. Christian Nordqvist, "Tamiflu May Not Be So Effective Against Bird Flu," Medical News Today, December 23, 2005, www.medicalnewstoday.com/healthnews.php?newsid=35339.

44. "Bird Flu Proving Resistant to Tamiflu Treatment," Associated Press and Reuters, December 22, 2005, www.msnbc.msn.com/id/10561923.

45. T. Jefferson, et al., "Anti-Virals for Influenza in Healthy Adults: Systemic Review,"

Lancet 367, no. 9507 (January 28, 2006): 303-13, www.ncbi.nlm.nih.gov/entrez/query.fcgi?cmd=Retrieve&db=PubMed&list_uids=16443037&dopt=Citation.

46. Sarah Boseley and Jonathan Watts, "Flu Drugs 'Will Not Work' If Pandemic Strikes," *Guardian*, January 19, 2005, www.guardian.co.uk/frontpage/story/0,,1689888,00.html.

47. Ibid.

48. "Outbreak! Tamiflu 'Useless' Against Avian Flu," World Net Daily, December 4 2005, www.worldnetdaily.com/news/article.asp?ARTICLE_ID=47725.

49. Ibid.

50. A. Moscona, "Neuraminidase Inhibitors for Influenza," *New England Journal of Medicine* 353 (2005): 363-73.

51. M. Kiso et al., "Resistant Influenza Virus in Children Treated with Oseltamivir: Descriptive Study," *Lancet* 364 (2004): 759-65.

52. R. R. Regoes and S. Bonhoeffer, "Emergence of Drug-Resistant Influenza Virus: Population Dynamical Considerations," *Science* 312, no. 5772 (April 21, 2006): 389-91.

53. "Health Canada Looking at Tamiflu Data After Reports of Deaths in Japan," Canadian Press, November 17, 2005, www.canada.com/health/story.html?id=d155eac6-df71-4639-a222-aee4d88f426c.

54. "FDA Probes Japan Deaths Possibly Linked to Tamiflu," *USA Today*, November 17, 2005, www.usatoday.com/news/health/2005-11-17-fda-tamiflu_x.htm.

55. "Regulatory Agency Asserts Tamiflu Safe," *USA Today*, November 19, 2005, www.usatoday.com/news/health/2005-11-19-tamiflu_x.htm.

56. "FDA Approves Tamiflu for Prevention of Influenza in Children under Age 12," press release, December 22, 2005 www.fda.gov/bbs/topics/news/2005/NEW01285.html.

57. Tamiflu Drug Information, www.fda.gov/cder/consumerinfo/druginfo/tamiflu.htm.

58. Tamiflu Drug Information. www.drugs.com/cons/Tamiflu.html.

59. Tamiflu (Oseltamivir Phosphate) Product Information: Roche Products Pty Ltd, 2005, www.rocheusa.com/products/tamiflu/pi.pdf.

60. Melissa M. Truffa, RPh, "One Year Post-Exclusivity Adverse Event Review for Tamiflu (Oseltamivir)," Pediatric Advisory Committee Meeting, November 18, 2005, http://www.fda.gov/ohrms/dockets/ac/05/slides/2005-4180s_03_truffa. ppt#256.

61. Christopher Ray, "No Panic—Dr. Stephan Lanka on Bird Flu, Vaccines, AIDS and the Corruption of Medicine," Factuell, October 27, 2005, www.faktuell.de/Hintergrund/Background367.shtml [in German], www.gnn.tv/A02138 [English translation].

62. Deborah MacKenzie, "Today's Bird Flu Vaccines Will Have to Do," *New Scientist* 2556 (June 16, 2006).

63. Interview with Ray Suarez, "Tracking the Bird Flu," March 2, 2006, www.pbs.org/newshour/bb/health/jan-june06/birdflu_3-02.html.

64. Sam Jaffe, "Clock Ticking on Vaccine Options," Wired, November 14, 2005, www.wired.com/news/medtech/0,1286,69556,00.html?tw=rss.TOP.

65. J.T. Macfarlane and W.S. Lim, "Bird Flu and Pandemic Flu," *BMJ* 331 (2005): 975-76, bmj.bmjjournals.com/cgi/content/full/331/7523/975.

66. "A Potential Influenza Pandemic: An Update on Possible Macroeconomic Effects and Policy Issues," Congressional Budget Office, May 22, 2006, www.cbo.gov/ftpdocs/72xx/doc7214/05-22-Avian%20Flu.pdf.

67. Barbara Loe Fisher, "Congress Set to Pass Law Eliminating Liability for Vaccine Injuries," National Vacine Information Center, press release, October 19, 2005, www. 909shot.com/PressReleases/ 101905Burrbill.htm.

68. "S.1873: A Bill to Prepare and Strengthen the Biodefenses of the United States Against Deliberate, Accidental, and Natural Outbreaks of Illness, and for Other Purposes," Introduced 10/17/2005, Senate Health, Education, Labor, and Pensions.

69. Barbara Loe Fisher, "Congress Set to Pass Law Eliminating Liability for Vaccine Injuries," National Vacine Information Center press release, October 19, 2005, www. 909shot.com/ PressReleases/101905Burrbill.htm.

70. Ibid.

71. Mike Adams, "The Lawlessness of the FDA, Big Pharma Immunity, and Crimes Against Humanity," News Target, June 29, 2006, www.newstarget.com/019497.html.

72. Gary Null, PhD, Carolyn Dean, MD, ND, Martin Feldman, MD, Debora Rasio, MD, and Dorothy Smith, PhD, "Death by Medicine," www.garynull.com, November 2003, www.garynull.com/documents/iatrogenic/deathbymedicine/ DeathByMedicine1. htm.

73. Eustace Mullins, *Murder by Injection*, The National Council for Medical Research, P. O. Box 1105, Staunton, Virginia 24401, 1988, 139.

74. Ibid., 139.

75. Jim Turner, personal communication with author.

76. Ibid.

77. Kristine Owram, "Specialist Warns Flu Pandemic Could Lead to Less Effective Vaccine Testing," Canadian Press, April 18, 2006, chealth.canoe.ca/channel_ health_news_details.asp?news_id=17477&news_channel_id=145&channel_id =145&relation_id=1555.

78. A. D. Langmuir, D. J. Bregman, L. T. Kurland, N. Nathanson, and M. Victor, "An Epidemiologic and Clinical Evaluation of Guillain-Barré Syndrome Reported in Association with the Administration of Swine Influenza Vaccines," Am J Epidemiol 119, no. 6 (1984): 841-79.

79. Gina Kolata, *Flu: The Story of the Great Influenza Pandemic* (CITY: Touchstone, 1999).

80. Laurie Garrett, "The Next Pandemic?" Foreign Affairs, July/August 2005, www. foreignaffairs.org/20050701faessay84401/laurie-garrett/the-next-pandemic.html.

81. "Achievements in Public Health, 1900-1999: Control of Infectious Diseases," *MMWR* 48, no. 29 (July 30, 1999): 621-29, www.cdc.gov/mmwr/preview/ mmwrhtml/mm4829a1.htm.

82. Ibid.

83. Harold Buttram, MD, "Vaccines Need a Closer Look," December 2, 2002, www.
mindfully.org/Health/2002/Vaccines-Unsafe20dec02.htm.
L. Dublin, "Health Progress, 1935–1945," New York: Metropolitan Life
Insurance Company, 1948, 12.

84. Bicentennial Edition: Historical Statistics of the United States, Colonial Times
to 1970, Part I, U.S. Department of Commerce, Bureau of the Census "Vital
Statistics and Health and Medical Care, Series B 149-166. U.S. Death Rate, for
Selected Causes: 1900 to 1970 Excluding Fetal Deaths." http://www2.census.gov/
prod2/statcom/documents/ct1970p1–03.pdf

85. Ibid.

86. "Achievements in Public Health, 1900–1999: Control of Infectious Diseases,"
Morbidity and Mortality Weekly Report 48, no. 29 (July 30, 1999): 621–29, www.cdc.
gov/mmwr/preview/ mmwrhtml/mm4829a1.htm.

87. "Age Adjusting to the 2000 Standard Population," American Cancer Society,
www.acsric.com/docroot/STT/content/STT_1_Age_Adjusted_Backgrounder.asp.

88. Robert S. Mendelsohn, *How to Raise a Healthy Child in Spite of Your Doctor*
(Chicago: Contemporary Books, March 1984).

89. Robert Mendelsohn, "The Medical Time Bomb of Immnuization Against
Disease," *East West Journal*, November 1984.

90. Eustace Mullins, *Murder by Injection*, The National Council for Medical
Research, P. O. Box 1105, Staunton, Virginia 24401, 1988, 132.

91. Ibid., 131–32.

92. Ibid., 132.

93. Ibid., 135.

94. Ibid., 138.

95. Ibid., 138.

96. Ibid., 133–34.

CHAPTER SIX

1. William Dufty, *Sugar Blues* (New York: Warner Books, 1975), 121.

2. Ibid., 132.

3. Loren Cordain, "Cereal Grains: Humanity's Double-Edged Sword," World Rev
Nutr Diet 84 (1999): 19–73.

4. "Doctors Fear Ontario Children May Not Live as Long as their Parents,"
Ontario Medical Association, October 4, 2005, www.oma.org/Media/news/
pr051004.asp.

5. O. Bermudez, "Consumption of Sweet Drinks Among American Adults from
the NHANES 1999–2000," Experimental Biology 2005, April 2–6, San Diego;
R. Murray, B. Frankowski, and H. Taras, "Are Soft Drinks a Scapegoat for
Childhood Obesity?" *Journal of Pediatrics* 146 (2005): 586.

6. "American Council on Exercise Recommends 60 Minutes of Physical Activity

a Day," news release, American Council on Exercise, September 16, 2002, www.acefitness.org/media/media_display.aspx?NewsID=143.

7. Marilyn C. Cornelis, BSc, Ahmed El-Sohemy, PhD, Edmond K. Kabagambe, PhD, Hannia Campos, PhD, "Coffee, CYP1A2 Genotype, and Risk of Myocardial Infarction," *JAMA* 295 (2006): 1135-41.

8. S. S. Tworoger, Y. Yasui, M. V. Vitiello, R. S. Schwartz, C. M. Ulrich, E. J. Aiello, M. L. Irwin, D. Bowen, J. D. Potter, and A. McTiernan, "Effects of a Yearlong Moderate-Intensity Exercise and a Stretching Intervention on Sleep Quality in Postmenopausal Women," *Sleep* 26, no. 7 (November 2003): 830-36.

9. Kathleen Fackelmann, "Stress Can Ravage the Body, Unless the Mind Says No," *USA Today*, March 21, 2005, www.usatoday.com/news/health/2005-03-21-stress_x.htm.

10. "Stress Management for the Health of It," National Ag Safety Database, Clemson Extension, www.cdc.gov/nasd/docs/d001201-d001300/d001245/d001245.html.

11. P. T. Liu, S. Stenger, H. Li et al., "Toll-Like Receptor Triggering of a Vitamin D-Mediated Human Antimicrobial Response," *Science* 311, no. 5768 (March 2006): 1770-73 [Epub February 2006].

12. M. T. Cantorna and B. D. Mahon, "D-hormone and the Immune System," J Rheumatol Suppl. 76 (September 2005): 11–20.

13. A. Zittermann, "Putting Cardiovascular Disease and Vitamin D Insufficiency into Perspective," *British Journal of Nutrition* 94, no. 4 (October 2005): 483–92.

14. K. L. Munger and S. M. Zhang, "Vitamin D Intake and Incidence of Multiple Sclerosis," *Neurology* 62, no. 1 (January 2004): 60–65.

15. L. C. Stene, G. Joner et al., "Use of Cod Liver Oil During the First Year of Life Is Associated with Lower Risk of Childhood-Onset Type 1 Diabetes: A Large, Population-Based, Case-Control Study," *American Journal of Clinical Nutrition* 78, no. 6 (December 2003): 1128–34.

16. M. T. Cantorna, C. Munsick , and C. Bemiss, "1,25-Dihydroxycholecalciferol Prevents and Ameliorates Symptoms of Experimental Murine Inflammatory Bowel Disease," J Nutr. 130, no. 11 (Novermber 2000): 2648–52.

17. L. A. Merlino, J. Curtis, T. R. Mikuls et al., "Vitamin D Intake Is Inversely Associated with Rheumatoid Arthritis: Results from the Iowa Women's Health Study," Arthritis Rheum. 50, no. 1 (January 2004): 72–77.

18. W. E.. Stumpf and T. H. Privette, "Light, Vitamin D and Psychiatry. Role of 1,25 Dihydroxyvitamin D3 (Soltriol) in Etiology and Therapy of Seasonal Affective Disorder and Other Mental Processes," *Psychopharmacology* (Berl) 97, no. 3 (1989): 285–94.

19. International Society for Developmental Neuroscience meeting in Sydney, Australia, February 2002.

20. Dr. Michael Holick, *The UV Advantage* (New York: I Books, May 2004).

21. H.S. Lim, R. Roychoudhuri, J. Peto, G. Schwartz, P. Baade, and H. Moller, "Cancer Survival Is Dependent on Season of Diagnosis and Sunlight Exposure," Int J Cancer, May 2, 2006 [Epub ahead of print].

22. Dr. David Feldman, *Vitamin D* (San Diego: Academic Press, 2004).

23. Sunlight, Nutrition and Health Research Center, summary of several research citations available at www.sunarc.org/papers.htm#chronic.

24. Dr. John Cannell, *The Vitamin D Newsletter*, June/July 2006, www.vitamindcouncil. com/newsletter/2006-june-july.shtml.

25. P. T. Liu et al., "Toll-Like Receptor Triggering of a Vitamin D-Mediated Human Antimicrobial Response," *Science* 311 no. 5768 (March 24, 2006): 1770-73 [Epub February 23, 2006].

26. Dr. John Cannell, *The Vitamin D Newsletter*, June/July 2006, www.vitamindcouncil. com/newsletter/2006-june-july.shtml.

    Cell Mol Biol (Noisy-le-grand) 49, no. 2 (March 2003): 277–300.

    J Immunol 173, no. 5 (September 1, 2004): 2909–12.

    FASEB J 19, no. 9 (July 2005): 1067–77.

    Science 311, no. 5768 (March 24, 2006): 1770–73.

27. Dr. John Cannell, *The Vitamin D Newsletter*, June/July 2006, www.vitamindcouncil. com/newsletter/2006-june-july.shtml.

28. E. K. Knott and V. K. Hancock, "Irradiated Blood Transfusion in Treatment of Infections," *Northwest Med.* 33 (1934): 200–204.

29. E. K. Knott, "Development of Ultraviolet Blood Irradiation," *American Journal of Surgery* 76, no. 2 (1948): 165–71.

30. K. Blunt and R. Cowan, *Ultraviolet Light and Vitamin D Nutrition* (Chicago: The University of Chicago Press, 1930).

31. G. P. Miley, "The Knott Technic of Ultraviolet Blood Irradiation in Acute Pyogenic Infections," *New York State Journal of Medicine* 42, no. 1 (1942): 38–46. G. P. Miley and J. A. Christensen, "Ultraviolet Blood Irradiation Therapy: Further Studies in Acute Infections," *American Journal of Surgery* 73 (1947): 486–93. E. W. Rebbeck, "Ultraviolet Irradiation of Auto-transfused Blood in the Treatment of Escherichia coli Septicemia," Archives of *Physical Therapy* 24 (1943): 158–67. F. E. Neff and C. M. Anderson, "Use of Ultraviolet Blood Irradiation in the Treatment of Bursitis and Tendinitis Calcarea," *American Journal of Surgery* 81, no. 6 (June 1951): 622–28. I. T. Schultz, "Use of the Knott Technic of Blood Irradiation Therapy in Cases of Threatened and Inevitable Abortion," *American Journal of Surgery* 88, no. 3 (September 1954): 421–24. R. C. Olney, "Treatment of Viral Hepatitis with the Knott Technic of Blood Irradiation," *American Journal of Surgery* 90, no. 3 (September 1955): 402–9.

32. "Mike Adams interviews Dr. Michael Holick, author of *The UV Advantage*," I Books, May 2004, www.quicktaninc.com/MichaelHolick.pdf.

33. Weston A. Price, DDS, *Nutrition and Physical Degeneration*, 6th Edition, Keats Publishing, Los Angeles, 1998.

34. Ron Schmid, ND, *The Untold Story of Milk* (Washington DC: New Trends Publishing, 2003).

35. William Dufty, *Sugar Blues* (New York: Warner Books, 1975).

36. Ibid., 109.

37. Ibid., 74.

38. Ibid., 110.

39. Ibid., 113.

40. Ibid., 110.

41. Sally Fallon, *Nourishing Traditions: The Cookbook That Challenges Politically Correct Nutrition and Diet Dictocrats* (Washington DC: New Trends Publishing, 2001), 95.

42. William Dufty, *Sugar Blues* (New York: Warner Books, 1975), 108.

43. Sally Fallon and Mary Enig, PhD, "The Scheme to Intervene, Caustic Commentary," Summer 2001, www.westonaprice.org/causticcommentary/cc2001su.html.

44. Barbara Demick, "Koreans' Kimchi Adulation, with a Side of Skepticism," *Los Angeles Times*, May 21, 2006, www.latimes.com/news/nationworld/world/la-fg-kimchi21may21,0,1528389,full.story?coll=la-home-headlines.

45. M. H. Jang, "South Korea, China in a Ferment Over Kimchi," Radio Free Asia, November 7, 2005, www.rfa.org/english/news/in_depth/2005/11/07/china_skor_kimchi/.

46. Mae-Wan Ho, "What Can You Believe About the Bird Flu?" Institute of Science in Society, May 18, 2006.

47. M. H. Jang. "South Korea, China in a Ferment Over Kimchi," Radio Free Asia, November 7, 2005, www.rfa.org/english/news/in_depth/2005/11/07/china_skor_kimchi/.

48. Dominique Patton, "Cabbage Dish Gaining Popularity as Flu-Fighter," Nutraingredients, November 16, 2005, www.nutraingredients.com/news/ng.asp?id=63932.

49. Y. J Oh, I. J Hwang, and C. Leitzmann, "Nutritional and Physiological Evaluation of *Kimchi*," The Science of *Kimchi*, Korean Society of Food Science and Technology, Seoul, 1994, 226, seafood.ucdavis.edu/iufost/lee.htm.

50. "Can Kimchi Sauerkraut Cure Avian Flu?" Axcess News, October 18, 2005, www.axcessnews.com/modules/wfsection/article.php?articleid=6183.

51. Dominique Patton, "Cabbage Dish Gaining Popularity as Flu-Fighter," Nutraingredients, November 16, 2005, www.nutraingredients.com/news/ng.asp?id=63932.

52. "Can Kimchi Sauerkraut Cure Avian Flu?" Axcess News, October 18, 2005, www.axcessnews.com/modules/wfsection/article.php?articleid=6183.

53. Sandor Ellix Katz, *Wild Fermentation* (Junction, VT: Chelsea Green Publishing Company, White River, 2003), 5.

54. Ibid., 5.

55. Ibid., 5.

56. Mike Battcock and Dr. Sue Azam-Ali, "Fermented Fruits and Vegetables. A Global Perspective," Food and Agriculture Organization of the United Nations, Rome, 1998, www.fao.org/docrep/x0560e/x0560e00.htm.

57. W. P Hammes and P. S. Tichaczek, "The Potential of Lactic-Acid Bacteria for the Production of Safe and Wholesome Food," Zeitschrift fur Lebenmitteltechnol, Germany, 1994.

58. B. J. B. Wood and M. M. Hodge, "Yeast Lactic Acid Bacteria Interaction," *Microbiology of Fermented Foods*, ed. B. J. B. Wood (UK: Elsevier Applied Science Publishers, 1985).

59. H. Matsusaki, K. Sonomoto, and A. Ishizaki, "Bacteriocins, Growth Inhibitory Substances of LacticAcid Bacteria," *Seibutsu Kogaku Kaishu Journal of the Society for Fermentation and Bioengineering*, Japan, 1997.

60. M. R Adams and L. Nicolaides, "Review of the Sensitivity of Different Foodborne Pathogens to Fermentation," Food Control, UK, 1997.

61. H. Gorama and L. B. Bullerman, "Antimycotic and Antiaflatoxigenic Effect of Lactic Acid Bacteria—a Review," *Journal of Food Protection*, 1995.

62. M. J. R. Nout, "Fungal Interactions in Food Fermentation," *Canadian Journal of Botany*, Canada, 1995.

63. G. Ottogalli, and A. Galli, *Fermented Foods in the Past and in the Future*, Annali di Microbiologia ed Enzimologia, Italy, 1997.

64. Y. Motarjemi, M. J. Nout, *Food Fermentation: A Safety and Nutrtional Assessment*, Bulletin of the World Health Organization, Switzerland, 1996.

65. R. H. Frohlich, M. Kunze, and I. Kiefer, "Cancer Preventive Impact of Naturally Occurring, Non-nutritive Constituents in Food," *Acta Medica Austriaca*, Austria, 1997.

66. K. H. Steinkraus, ed. *Handbook of Indigenous Fermented Foods* (New York: Marcel Dekker, Inc., 1995).

67. Andre G. van Veen and Keith H. Steinkraus, "Nutritive Value and Wholesomeness of Fermented Foods," *Agricultural and Food Chemistry* 18, no. 4 (1970): 576.

68. Watson, F.E., Ngesa, A., Onyango, J., Alnwick, D. and Tomkins, A.M., "Fermentation—A Traditional Anti-Diarrheal Practice Lost," *International Journal of Food Sciences and Nutrition*, 1996.

69. B. Svanberg, *Fermentation of Cereals: Traditional Household Technology with Nutritional Benefits for Young Children*, IDRC Currents 2, Canada, 1992.

70. Sally Fallon, *Nourishing Traditions: The Cookbook that Challenges Politically Correct Nutrition and the Diet Dictocrats* (Washington DC: New Trends Publishing, 2001), 509.

71. P. A. Barrett, E. Beveridge, P. L. Bradley et al., "Biological Activities of Some Alpha-dithiosemicarbazones," *Nature* 206, no. 991 (June 1965): 1340–41.

72. M. Tolonen, M. Taipale, B. Viander, J. M. Pihlava, H. Korhonen, and E. L.

Ryhanen,. "Plant-Derived Biomolecules in Fermented Cabbage," *J. Agric. Food Chem.* 50, no. 23 (2002): 6798-6803. DOI: 10.1021/jf0109017.

73. U. Svanberg et al., "Bioavailability of Iron in Lactic Fermented Foods," in *Processing and Quality of Foods*, eds. P. Zeuthen et al., vol. 2, 116–21. Elsevier Applied Science Publishers, London, 1990.

74. "Dietary Reference Intakes: Thiamin, Riboflavin, Niacin, Vitamin B-6, Vitamin B-12, Pantothenic Acid, Biotin, and Choline," Institute of Medicine, Food and Nutrition Board, Washington DC: National Academy Press, 1998, 390–422.

75. S. Gilman, R. A. Koeppe, R. D. Chervin, F. B. Consens, R. Little, H. An, L. Junck, and M. Heumann, "REM Sleep Behavior Disorder Is Related to Striatal Monoaminergic Deficit in MSA," *Neurology* 61 (July 2003): 29–34.

     S. Gilman, R. D. Chervin, R. A. Koeppe, F.B. Consens, R. Little, H. An, L. Junck, and M. Heumann, "Obstructive Sleep Apnea Is Related to a Thalamic Cholinergic Deficit in MSA," *Neurology* 61 (July 2003): 35–39.

76. Annelies Schoneck and Klaus Kaufmann, *The Cultured Cabbage* (Vancouver: Alive Books, 1997).

77. N. S. Tropskaya, T. S. Popova, and G. I. Soloveva, "Effect of Drugs with Various Mechanisms of Action on Propulsive Activity of the Small Intestine," *Bull Exp Biol Med* 140, no. 3 (September 2005): 268–70.

78. "Atopy in Children of Families with an Anthroposophical Lifestyle," *Lancet* 353, no. 9163 (May 1, 1999): 1485–88.

79. Ibid.

80. M. Tolonen, M. Taipale, B. Viander, J. M. Pihlava, H. Korhonen, and E. L. Ryhanen, "Plant-Derived Biomolecules in Fermented Cabbage," *J. Agric. Food Chem.* 50, no. 23 (2002): 6798-6803. DOI: 10.1021/jf0109017

81. Ibid.

82. D. R. Pathak et al., "Joint Association of High Cabbage/Sauerkraut Intake at 12–13 Years of Age and Adulthood with Reduced Breast Cancer Risk in Polish Migrant Women: Results from the US Component of the Polish Women's Health Study," Abstract number 3697, presented at the AACR 4th Annual Conference on Frontiers in Cancer Prevention Research, October 30–November 2, 2005, Baltimore, Maryland.

83. U. Preiss et al., "Effect of Fermentation on Components of Vegetable," *Deutsche Lebensmittel-Rundschau* 98, no. 11 (2002): 400–5.

84. Kaayla T. Daniel, *The Whole Soy Story* (Washington DC: New Trends Publishing, 2005).

85. B. Kovac, *The Use of the Mould Rhizopus oligosporus in Food Production*, Food Technology and Biology, 1997.

86. O. Parades-Lopez, *Nutrition and Safety Considerations in Applications of Biotechnology to Traditional Fermented Foods*, report of an Ad Hoc Panel of the Board on Science and Technology for International Development, National Academy Press, Washington DC, USA, 1992.

87. H. Liljeberg and I. Bjo¨rck I "Bioavailability of Starch in Bread Products. Postprandial Glucose and Insulin Responses in Healthy Subjects and In Vitro Resistant Starch Content," *European Journal of Clinical Nutrition* 48 (1994): 151–63.

88. H. G. Liljeberg, C. H. Lonner, and I. M. Bjorck, "Sourdough Fermentation or Addition of Organic Acids or Aorresponding Salts to Bread Improves Nutritional Properties of Starch in Healthy Humans," *Journal of Nutrition* 125, no. 6 (June 1995): 1503–11.

89. Sally Fallon, *Nourishing Traditions* (Washington: New Trends Publishing, 2001), 455.

90. H. S. Gill, "Stimulation of the Immune System by Lactic Cultures," Intl. Dairy Journal 8 (1998): 535–44.

91. H. S. Gill, "Potential of Using Dietary Lactic Acid Bacteria for Enhancement of Immunity," *Dialogue* 32 (1999): 6–11.

92. J. W. Lee, J. G. Shin, E. H. Kim, H. E. Kang, I. B. Yim, J. Y. Kim, H. G. Joo, and H. J. Woo, "Immunomodulatory and Antitumor Effects In Vivo by the Cytoplasmic Fraction of Lactobacillus casei and Bifidobacterium longum," *Journal of Veterinary Science* 5, no. 1 (March 2004): 41–48.

93. B. A. Friend et al., "Nutritional and Therapeutic Aspects of Lactobacilli," *Journal of Applied Nutrition* 36, no. 2 (1984): 125–53.

94. C. F. Fernandes et al., "Therapeutic Role of Dietary Lactobacilli and Lactobacillus Fermented Dairy Products," *Fed of Eur Microbiol Rev* 46 (1987): 343–56.

95. G. Perdigon, E. Vintini, S. Alvarez, M. Medina, and M. Medici, "Study of the Possible Mechanisms Involved in the Mucosal Immune System Activation by Lactic Acid Bacteria," *Journal of Dairy Science* 82 (1999): 1108–14.

96. S. Salminen, C. Bouley, and M. C. Boutron Ruault, "Functional Food Science and Gastrointestinal Physiology and Function," 1Br. J. Nutr. 80 (1998): 147–71.

97. Y. J Kim and R. H. Liu, "Increase of Conjugated Linoleic Acid Content in Milk by Fermentation with Lactic Acid Bacteria," *Journal of Food Science* 67 (2002): 1731-37.

98. Mike Battcock and Dr. Sue Azam-Ali, "Fermented Fruits and Vegetables: A Global Perspective," Food and Agriculture Organization of the United Nations, Rome ,1998, www.fao.org/docrep/x0560e/x0560e00.htm.

99. Sally Fallon, *Nourishing Traditions: The Cookbook That Challenges Politically Correct Nutrition and the Diet Dictocrats* (Washington DC: New Trends Publishing, 2001), 509.

100. K. M. Shahani and R. C. Chandan, "Nutritional and Healthful Aspects of Cultured and Culture-Containing Dairy Foods," *Journal of Dairy Science* 62, no. 10 (October 1979): 1685-94.

101. C. F. Fernandes, K. M. Shahani, and M. A. Amer, "Therapeutic Role of Dietary Lactobacilli and Lactobacillic Fermented Dairy Products," *FEMS Microbiology Reviews* 46, no. 3 (1987).

102. "Yogurt for a Longer :ife," The World's Healthiest Foods, The George Mateljan Foundation, www.whfoods.com/genpage.php?tname=foodspice&dbid=124.

103. Ripudaman S. Beniwal, Vincent C. Arena, Leno Thomas, Sudhir Narla, Thomas F. Imperiale, Rauf A. Chaudhry, and Usman A. Ahmad, "A Randomized Trial of Yogurt for Prevention of Antibiotic-Associated Diarrhea," *Digestive Diseases and Sciences* 48, no. 10 (October 2003): 2077–82.

104. G. Boudraa, M. Touhami, P. Pochart, R. Soltana, J. Y. Mary, and J. F. Desjeux, "Effect of Feeding Yogurt Versus Milk in Children with Persistent Diarrhea," J. Pediatr Gastroenerol Nutr 11, no. 4 (November 1990): 509–12.

105. Nobuko Maeda, professor of microbiology, Tsurumi University, Yokohama, Japan, and Bruce J. Paster, PhD., senior staff member, department of molecular genetics, The Forsythe Institute, Boston, presentation, International Association for Dental Research meeting, Baltimore, March 10, 2005.

106. Jennifer Warner, "Yogurt: An Antidote to Bad Breath," MedicineNet.com, March 10, 2005, onhealth.webmd.com/script/main/art.asp?articlekey=56032.

107. Julio Villena, Silvia Racedo, Graciela Aguero, Elena Bru, Marcela Medina, and Susana Alvarez, "Lactobacillus Casei Improves Resistance to Pneumococcal Respiratory Infection in Malnourished Mice," *The American Society for Nutritional Sciences, Journal of Nutrition* 135 (June 2005): 1462-69.

108. Simin Nikbin Meydani and Woel-Kyu Ha, "Immunologic Effects of Yogurt," *American Journal of Clinical Nutrition* 71, no. 4 (April 2000): 861-72.

109. Natasha Trenev, *Probiotics: Nature's Internal Healers* (New York: Avery, 1998).

110. A. Cevikbas, E. Yemni, F. W. Ezzedenn, and T. Yardimici, "Antitumoural, Antibacterial and Antifungal Activities of Kefir and Kefir Grain," Phytother. Res. 8 (1994): 78–82.

111. N. Furukawa, A. Matsuoka, and Y. Yamanaka, "Effects of Orally Administered Yogurt and Kefir on Tumor Growth in Mice," J. Japan. Soc. Nutr. Food Sci. 43 (1990): 45053.

112. N. Furukawa, A. Matsuoka, T. Takahashi, and Y. Yamanaka, "Effects of Fermented Milk on the Delayed-Type Hypersensitivity Response and Survival day in Mice Bearing Meth-A," Anim. Sci. Tec 62 (1991): 579–85.

113. W. Kneifel and H. K. Mayer, "Vitamin profiles of kefirs made from milks of different species," *International Journal of Food Science & Technology* 26 (1991): 423–28.

114. Semih Otes and Ozem Cagindi, "Kefir: A Probiotic Dairy-Composition, Nutritional and Therapeutic Aspects," *Pakistan Journal of Nutrition* 2, no. 2 (2003): 54–59.

115. Ibid.

CHAPTER·SEVEN

1. John Ikerd, "The High Cost of Cheap Food," *Small Farm Today*, July/August 2001.

2. "The Market for Organic Foods," FAQS.org, www.faqs.org/nutrition/Ome-Pop/Organic-Foods.html.

3. "Demand for Organic Food Outstrips Supply," *Forbes*, July 6, 2006, www.forbes. com/work/feeds/ap/2006/07/06/ap2862437.html.

4. National Research Council, Committee on Scientific and Regulatory Issues Underlying Pesticide Use Patterns and Agricultural Innovation, "Regulating Pesticides in Food: the Delaney Paradox, Executive Summary," 1987.

5. Ewa Rembialkowska, "Organic Food Quality—Axioms and Ambiguities," paper presented at Joint Organic Congress, Odense, Denmark, May 30–31, 2006, orgprints.org/7594/01/Odense_Congress-2006_3_II_2006.doc.

6. S. B. Kramer, J. P. Reganold, J. D. Glover, B. J. M. Bohannan, and H. A. Mooney, "Reduced Nitrate Leaching and Enhanced Denitrifier Activity and Efficiency in Organically Fertilized Soils," Proceedings of the National Academy of Sciences (PNAS), March 2006.

7. Ibid.

8. Chuck Benbrook, PhD, "Breaking the Mold—Impacts of Organic and Conventional Farming Systems on Mycotoxins in Food and Livestock Feed," Organic Center for Education and Promotion, September 2005.

9. Dr. Chuck Benbrook, personal communication with author

10. Dr. Chuck Benbrook, personal communication with author

11. M. E. Olsson, C. S. Andersson, S. Oredsson, R. H. Berglund, and K. E. Gustavsson, "Antioxidant Levels and Inhibition of Cancer Cell Proliferation In Vitro by Extracts from Organically and Conventionally Cultivated Strawberries," J Agric Food Chem 54, no. 4 (2006): 1248–55.

12. S. Y. Wang, R. Feng, Y. Lu, L. Bowman, and M. Ding, "Inhibitory Effect on Activator Protein-1, Nuclear Factor-kappaB, and Cell Transformation by Extracts of Strawberries (Fragaria x ananassa Duch.)," J Agric Food Chem 53, no. 10 (2005): 4187–93.

13. B. Rekha, S. Naik, and R. Prasad, "Pesticide Residues in Organic and Conventional Food—Risk analysis,"Chemical Health and Safety in press doi:10.1016/j.chs.2005.01.012.

14. C. Lu, K. Toepel, R. Irish, R. A. Fenske, D. B. Barr, and R. Bravo, "Organic Diets Significantly Lower Children's Dietary Exposure to Organophosphorus Pesticides," *Environ Health Perspect* 114, no. 2 (2006): 260–63.

15. Ewa Rembialkowska, "Organic Food Quality—Axioms and Ambiguities," paper presented at Joint Organic Congress, Odense, Denmark, May 30–31, 2006. orgprints.org/7594/01/Odense_Congress-2006_3_II_2006.doc

16. Ibid.

17. c. Ip, J. A. Scimeca et al., "Conjugated Linoleic Acid. A Powerful Anticarcinogen from Animal Fat Sources," *Cancer* 74, no. 3, suppl. (1994): 1050–54.

18. A. Aro, S. Mannisto, I. Salminen, M. L. Ovaskainen, V. Kataja, and M. Uusitupa, "Inverse Association Between Dietary and Serum Conjugated Linoleic Acid and Risk of Breast Cancer in Postmenopausal Women," *Nutrition and Cancer* 38, no. 2 (2000): 151–57.

19. P. Bougnonx, F. Lavillonniere, E. Riboli, et al. "Inverse Relationship between CLA in Adipose Breat Tissue and Risk of Breast Cancer.: A case-control study in France. Am. Oil Chemists' Meeting, 1999 [Abstract]. *Health and Nutrition*, section 3, 543

20. Used with permission from Environmental Working Group, Shopper's Guide to Pesticides in Produce, www.FoodNews.org or www.walletguide.org.

21. "Acrylamide (CASRN 79-06-1) Integrated Risk Information System," www.epa.gov/iris/subst/0286.htm.

22. "Opinion of the Scientific Committee on Food on New Findings Regarding the Presence of Acrylamide in Food," European Commission, July 3, 2002, ec.europa.eu/food/fs/sc/scf/out131_en.pdf.

23. Peter W. B. Phillips, "Policy, National Regulation, and International Standards for GM Foods," Biotechnology and Genetics Resource Policies, International Food Policy Resource Institute, January 2003.

24. Craig Winters personal communication with author.

25. Ibid,

26. Peter W. B. Phillips, "Policy, National Regulation, and International Standards for GM Foods," Biotechnology and Genetics Resource Policies, International Food Policy Resource Institute, January 2003.

27. Mae-Wan Ho and Lim Li Ching; *GMO Free: Exposing the Hazards of Biotechnology to Ensure the Integrity of Our Food Supply* (Ridgefield: Vital Health Publishing, 2004).

28. "US Genetic Contamination of Organic Produce Pervades the World," Weekly International News from Organic Trade, May 3, 2001.

29. Dr. Bruce Griffin and Dr. A. Lee, "Dietary Cholesterol, Eggs and Coronary Heart Disease Risk in Perspective," Centre for Nutrition & Food Safety, School of Biomedical & Molecular Sciences, University of Surrey, UK, March 2006, www.marketwire.com/mw/release_html_b1?release_id=130750.

30. Ibid.

31. Ibid.

32. "Egg Trivia: All You Ever Need to Know," The Egg Nutrition Center, www.enc-online.org/trivia.htm.

33. "A Brief History of Eggs," Canadian Egg Marketing Agency, www.canadaegg.ca/bins/content_page.asp?cid=6-63&lang=1.

34. A. Tolan, J. Robertson, C. R. Orton, M. J. Head, A. A. Christie and B. A. Millburn, "Studies on the Composition of Food: 5. The Chemical Composition of Eggs Produced under Battery, Deep Litter and Free Range Conditions," Br J Nutr. 31, no. 2 (March 1974): 185–200.

35. J. Schlatterer and D. E. Breithaupt, "Xanthophylls in Commercial Egg Yolks," *Journal of Agriculture and Food Chemistry* 54 (2006): 2267–73.

36. Linda E. Kelemen, James R. Cerhan, Unhee Lim, Scott Davis, Wendy Cozen, Maryjean Schenk, Joanne Colt, Patricia Hartge, and Mary H. Ward, "Vegetables, Fruit, and Antioxidant-Related Nutrients and Risk of Non-

Hodgkin Lymphoma: A National Cancer Institute–Surveillance, Epidemiology, and End Results Population-Based Case-Control Study," *American Journal of Clinical Nutrition* 83 (June 2006): 1401–10.

37. B. K Hope, R. Baker, E. D. Edel, A. T. Hogue, W. D. Schlosser, R. Whiting R, M. McDowell, and R. A. Morales, "An Overview of the Salmonella Enteritidis Risk Assessment for Shell Eggs and Egg Products," *Risk Anal.* 22, no. 2 (April 2002): 203–18.

38. Sir Albert Howard, *An Agricultural Testament* (London: Oxford University Press, 1943).

39. Country of Origin Labeling, 2002 Farm Bill Provisions, www.ams.usda.gov/COOL/.

40. "Whole Foods Pledges Greater Support of Small Farms," Reuters, June 30, 2006, today.reuters.com/stocks/QuoteCompanyNewsArticle.aspx?view=CN& storyID=2006-06-30T220250Z_01_N30307245_RTRIDST_0_FOOD-LOCAL-WHOLEFOODS.XML&rpc=66.

41. Michael Pollan, *The Omnivore's Dilemma: A Natural History of Four Meals* (New York: The Penguin Press, 2006), 139.

42. New Penn, "Campaign Helps Shoppers Find Local Goods," *Progressive Grocer*, July 5, 2006, www.progressivegrocer.com/progressivegrocer/magazine/article_display.jsp?vnu_content_id=1002765335.

43. Rich Pirog and Andrew Benjamin, "Checking the Food Odometer: Comparing Food Miles for Local Versus Conventional Produce Sales to Iowa Institutions," Leopold Center for Sustainable Agriculture, Iowa State University, July 2003, www.leopold.iastate.edu/pubs/staff/files/food_travel072103.pdf.

44. Ibid.

45. Ibid.

46. Ibid.

47. William D. Heffernan, PhD, and Mary K. Hendrickson, PhD, "Multi-National Concentrated Food Processing and Marketing Systems and the Farm Crisis," presented at the Annual Meeting of the American Association for the Advancement of Science, Boston, MA, February 14–19, 2002; Symposium: "Science and Sustainability; the Farm Crisis: How the Heck Did We Get Here?"

48. "Jerry Kay Interview with Michael Pollan, author of *The Omnivore's Dilemma*," Beyond Organic, April 19, 2006, www.beyondorganic.com/shows/beyondorganic 041906.mp3.

49. Ibid.

50. "A History of American Agriculture, 1776–1990," inventors.about.com/library/inventors/blfarm4.htm.

51. Parija Bhatnagar, "Wal-Mart's Next Conquest: Organics," *CNN Money.com*, May 1, 2006, money.cnn.com/2006/05/01/news/companies/walmart_organics/index.htm.

52. Hedrick Smith and Rick Young, "Is Wal-Mart Good for America?" *Frontline*, November 16, 2004.

53. Bill Heffernan, personal communication with author.

54. John Ikerd, "The High Cost of Cheap Food," *Small Farm Today*, July/August 2001

55. Jo Robinson, "Growing Corn and Soy Causes Six Times More Soil Erosion Than Pasture," www.eatwild.com/ReadMore10.htm.

56. "Pasture Reduces Topsoil Erosion by 93 Percent," chart courtesy of Jo Robinson, www.eatwild.com/ReadMore13.htm.

57. Robert P. Stone and Neil Moore, "Control of Soil Erosion," Ontario Ministry of Agriculture, Food and Rural Affairs, January 1996, www.omafra.gov.on.ca/english/engineer/ facts/95-089.htm.

58. "Study Shows Dairies Reduce Soil Erosion," Dairy Herd Management staff, Dairy Herd Management, January 13, 2004, www.dairyherd. com/directories.asp?pgID= 724&ed_id=3159&component_id=871,

59. "Growing Corn and Soy Causes Six Times More Soil Erosion Than Pasture," chart courtesy of Jo Robinson, www.eatwild.com/ReadMore10.htm.

60. "Farmers Market Growth, 1994–2004," USDA, www.ams.usda.gov/farmers markets/FarmersMarketGrowth.htm.

61. Ibid.

62. Harold Brubaker, "Fresh, Local and Growing," *Philly News*, May 30, 2006, www.philly.com/mld/inquirer/business/14695520.htm.

63. Ibid.

64. Brian Moyer. personal communication with author.

65. Joel Salatin, *Holy Cows & Hog Heaven* (Swoope, VA: Polyface Inc., 2004), 105.

66. Ibid.

67. Ibid.

68. John Ikerd, "The High Cost of Cheap Food," *Small Farm Today*, July/August 2001.

69. Lee Ann Cox and Kevin Foley, "Fresh Voices from the Vermont Fresh Network," *Vermont Commons*, Issue 6, October 2005, vtcommons.org/node/218.

70. Ibid.

71. Ibid.

72. Alternative Farming Systems Information Center, Community Supported Agriculture (CSA), http://www.nal.usda.gov/afsic/csa/.

73. Food Circles Networking Project, University of Missouri Extension, Connecting Farmers, Consumers and Communities, http://foodcircles.missouri.edu/

74. Food Circles Networking Project, University of Missouri Extension, Connecting Farmers, Consumers and Communities, http://foodcircles.missouri.edu/vision.htm.

75. "What Is the Leopold Center," The Leopold Center, www.leopold.iastate.edu/about/leopoldcenter.htm.

76. The Ohio State University Extension, *Amazing Graze News*, forages.osu.edu/News/Archive/2003/amazegrazejan03.html.

77. "Welcome to Appalachian Farming Systems Research Center," The United

States Department of Agriculture, Agricultural Research Service, www.ars.usda. gov/Main/site_main.htm?modecode=19-32-00-00.

78. "Public Health Association Calls for Moratorium on Factory Farms; Cites Health Issues, Pollution," Johns Hopkins Bloomberg School of Public Health, press release, January 9, 2004, www.jhsph.edu/publichealthnews/press_releases/ PR_2004/farm_moratorium.html.

79. Ibid.

80. Ibid.

81. Ibid.

82. Ibid.

83. John Ikerd, "The High Cost of Cheap Food," *Small Farm Today*, July/August 2001.

84. James Roth, DVM, PhD, "Safeguarding American Agriculture from Foreign Animal Diseases, Center for Food Security and Public Health," Iowa State University, 2004, www.cfsph.iastate.edu/TrainTheTrainer/ppts/pptSafeguarding. ppt#682,3,Vulnerabilities.

CHAPTER EIGHT

1. Michael Brower, PhD, and Warren Leon, PhD, *The Consumer's Guide to Effective Environmental Choices: Practical Advice from the Union of Concerned Scientists* (New York: Three Rivers Press, 1999).

APPENDIX

Recipes

Sauerkraut

Courtesy of Sally Fallon, *Nourishing Traditions*, page 92
(Makes 1 quart)

1	medium cabbage, cored and shredded
1	tablespoon caraway seeds
1	tablespoon sea salt
4	tablespoons whey[1] (if not available, use an additional 1 tablespoon salt)

In a bowl, mix cabbage with caraway seeds, sea salt and whey*. Pound with a wooden pounder or a meat hammer for about 10 minutes to release juices. Place in a quart-sized, wide-mouth mason jar and press down firmly with a pounder or meat hammer until juices come to the top of the cabbage. The top of the cabbage should be at least 1 inch below the top of the jar. Cover tightly and keep at room temperature for about 3 days before transferring to cold storage. The sauerkraut may be eaten immediately, but it improves with age.

---

*Whey is a wonderful starter culture that you can buy from a local farmer. Otherwise, when you make your own yogurt (or a yogurt with live bacteria), line a strainer with a clean dish towel, pour in the yogurt, and let stand for several hours. The whey will run into a bowl underneath and the milk solids will stay in the strainer.

Yogurt

Courtesy of Sandor Ellix Katz, *Wild Fermentation*, pages 76-77
(Makes 1 quart)

You need a starter culture to make yogurt. You can buy spe-
cialized cultures for this, or use any live-culture yogurt. If you use
the latter, make sure the yogurt says "Contains live cultures" on the
label; otherwise, it has probably been pasteurized, which kills the
bacteria. Once you make your first batch, save a little yogurt from
each batch to start the next one. With regular attention, a starter
culture can keep on going indefinitely.

Timeframe: 8 to 24 hours

Special Equipment
    Quart jar
    Insulated cooler

Ingredients

1   quart whole milk (be sure to use raw milk)
1   tablespoon fresh live-culture plain yogurt for starter
        culture

1. Preheat the jar and insulated cooler with hot water so they will
   not drain heat from the yogurt and it can stay warm to ferment.

2. Heat the milk until bubbles begin to form. If you use a ther-
   mometer, heat milk to 180° F. Use gentle heat, and stir frequently,
   to avoid burning the milk. It does not need to come to a full boil.
   The heating is not absolutely necessary, but it results in a thicker
   yogurt.

3. Cool the milk to 110° F, or the point where it feels hot, but it is
   not hard to keep your (clean!) finger in it. You can speed up the

cooling process by setting the pot with hot milk into a bowl or pot of cold water. Don't let the milk get too cool; the yogurt cultures are most active in the above-body-temperature range.

4. Mix starter yogurt into the milk. Use just 1 tablespoon per quart. Mix the starter thoroughly into the milk, and pour the mixture into the preheated jar.

5. Cap the jar and place it in the preheated insulated cooler. If much space remains in the cooler, fill it with hot water bottles (not too hot to touch) and/or towels. Close the cooler. Place the cooler in a warm spot where it will not be disturbed.

6. Check the yogurt after 8 to 12 hours. It should have a tangy flavor and some thickness. If it isn't thick, warm it up by filling the insulated cooler with hot water around the jar of yogurt, adding more starter, and leaving it 4 to 8 more hours. You can leave it to ferment longer if you wish. It will become more sour, as more of the milk's lactose is converted into lactic acid. A longer fermentation period can often make yogurt digestible even for lactose intolerant individuals.

7. Yogurt can store in the refrigerator for weeks, though its flavor will become more sour over time. Save some of your yogurt to use as starter for the next batch.

Kefir

from *Wild Fermentation*, pages 79-81
(makes 1 quart)

Kefir is made with "grains", actually colonies of beneficial yeast and bacteria that look like curds, which you can strain out after fermentation, then use for your next batch. Kefir grains are available online or from health food stores.

Timeframe: Days

Ingredients:

1   quart milk (be sure to use raw milk!)
1   tablespoon kefir grains

Process:

1. Fill a jar with milk, no more than two-thirds full. Add kefir grains, and cap.

2. Leave at room temperature for 24-48 hours, agitating jar periodically. Milk will become bubbly, then coagulate and separate. You can remix it by shaking.

3. Strain out the grains with any straining implement. You may need to use a spoon or chopstick (or your clean finger) to stir and keep the strainer from clogging up with grains. Grains will grow and multiply in number over time. You only need a tablespoon or so of grains to keep your kefir going. You can eat the extras, toss them in the compost, give them away to your friends, or use them to try culturing other things. Kefir grains are very versatile.

4. Enjoy your kefir, and use the grains to start another batch. Kefir can stay out at room temperature and continue to develop, or it can be refrigerated. If you tighten the lid on a jar of fermenting kefir, it will develop effervescence.

ABOUT THE AUTHOR

DR. JOSEPH MERCOLA is an osteopathic physician who is board-certified by the American College Osteopathic General Practitioners in family medicine. His goals are to help people be as healthy as possible by (1) providing the health and medical knowledge and resources of most benefit, and (2) exposing the corporate, government, and mass-media hype that diverts people away from what is truly best for their health and often sends them straight into an early grave.

Dr. Mercola received his Medical degree from Midwestern University, formerly the Chicago College of Osteopatric Medicine He is a member of the Association of American Physicians and Surgeons. He has frequently been interviewed on national and local news, including ABC's *World News Tonight with Peter Jennings,* CNN, CBS, NBC, and ABC local news shows, and dozens of nationally broadcast radio shows. Dr. Mercola's Web site, www.Mercola.com, is the most visited natural health site on the Internet.

PAM KILLEEN is an Investigative Reporter who has been independently studying nutrition and natural health for twenty years. Pam's interest in nutrition and natural health stems from overcoming a lengthy battle with chronic fatigue, fibromyalgia, multiple chemical sensitivities and environmental illness. Through her experience, she understands why consumers are so confused about what to do to achieve optimal health. The focus of her work is to expose just how very sophisticated propaganda prevents people from learning the truth about health and nutrition and covers stories and interviews that would normally be ignored by the corporately controlled media. Pam believes it is important to balance stories and interviews by offering practical solutions to the many problems we are facing today.

Take the Test Designed by Dr. Mercola to Discover How Strong *Your* Immune System Actually Is for FREE Right Now!

Just go to www.GreatBirdFluHoax.com to Take Your FREE Test . . . You Will Get Your Personal "Immunity Score" & Disease Prevention Advice <u>Instantly</u>!

As this book demonstrates, your worries should not be focused on a bird flu pandemic.

However, you **should** definitely be concerned about the strength of your immune system, because there are multiple disease epidemics currently raging that are *very* REAL. This includes cancer, heart disease, diabetes, Alzheimer's and more—and your immune system is your ONE and ONLY real line of defense against them.

Furthermore, on the remote chance that a bird flu pandemic actually occurred, if you had a healthy immune system your body would easily be able to defend you against it naturally . . . no vaccines or other drugs required!

As a *Great Bird Flu Hoax* reader, you are strongly encouraged to take the new free test designed by Dr. Mercola to get a solid idea of how strong your immune system really is. When you take this free test at GreatBirdFluHoax.com you will get:

- **Your immune system strength results instantly,** with some key insights on what you can do to start improving your immune system today

- **A FREE subscription to Dr. Mercola's "eHealthy News You Can Use" newsletter** — now the world's #1 health newsletter with over 600,000 subscribers. You'll get insider insights from top experts to keep improving your immune system… so you don't have to worry about chronic diseases (or hype like the bird flu) anymore

Go to www.GreatBirdFluHoax.com for Your FREE Immune System Test Right Now!